C - Can't say you are healthy without getting checked.

O - Only smart people get checked.

L - Let's all go get checked.

O - Oy vey... go get checked.

N - Now! Go get checked now!

O - Oh boy, I hope you are getting checked.

S - Seriously, go get checked.

C - Can someone please think about the children?

O - Oh my, this word has lots of Os.

P - Please go get checked.

Y - Y? Because it is smart to get checked.

Colonoscopy, colonoscopy
The day is finally coming.
My 40s have been fun,
Now it's time to check
my plumbing!

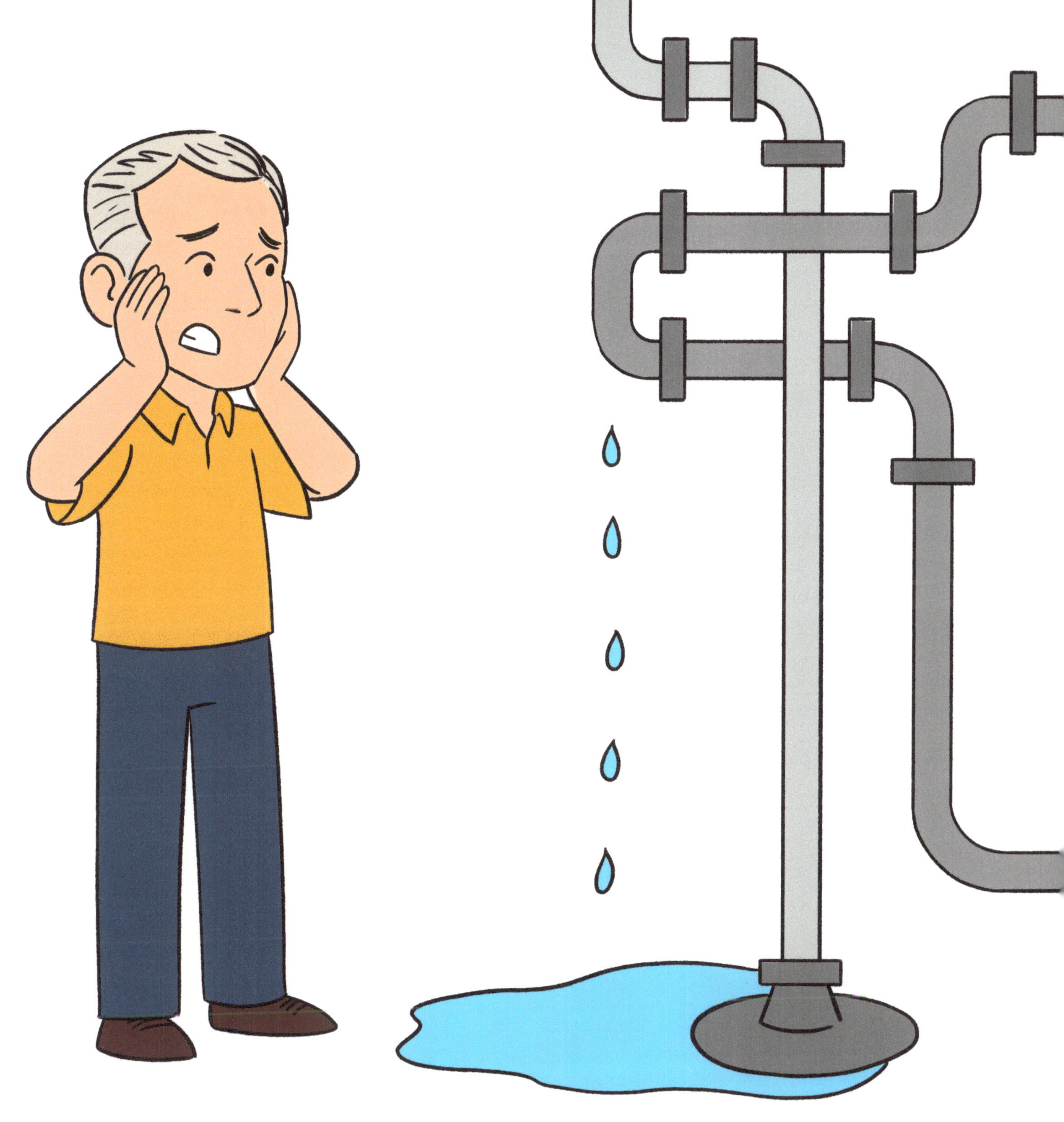

Getting older has its perks,
And also its set-backs.
Like having a stranger,
Probe in my butt crack.

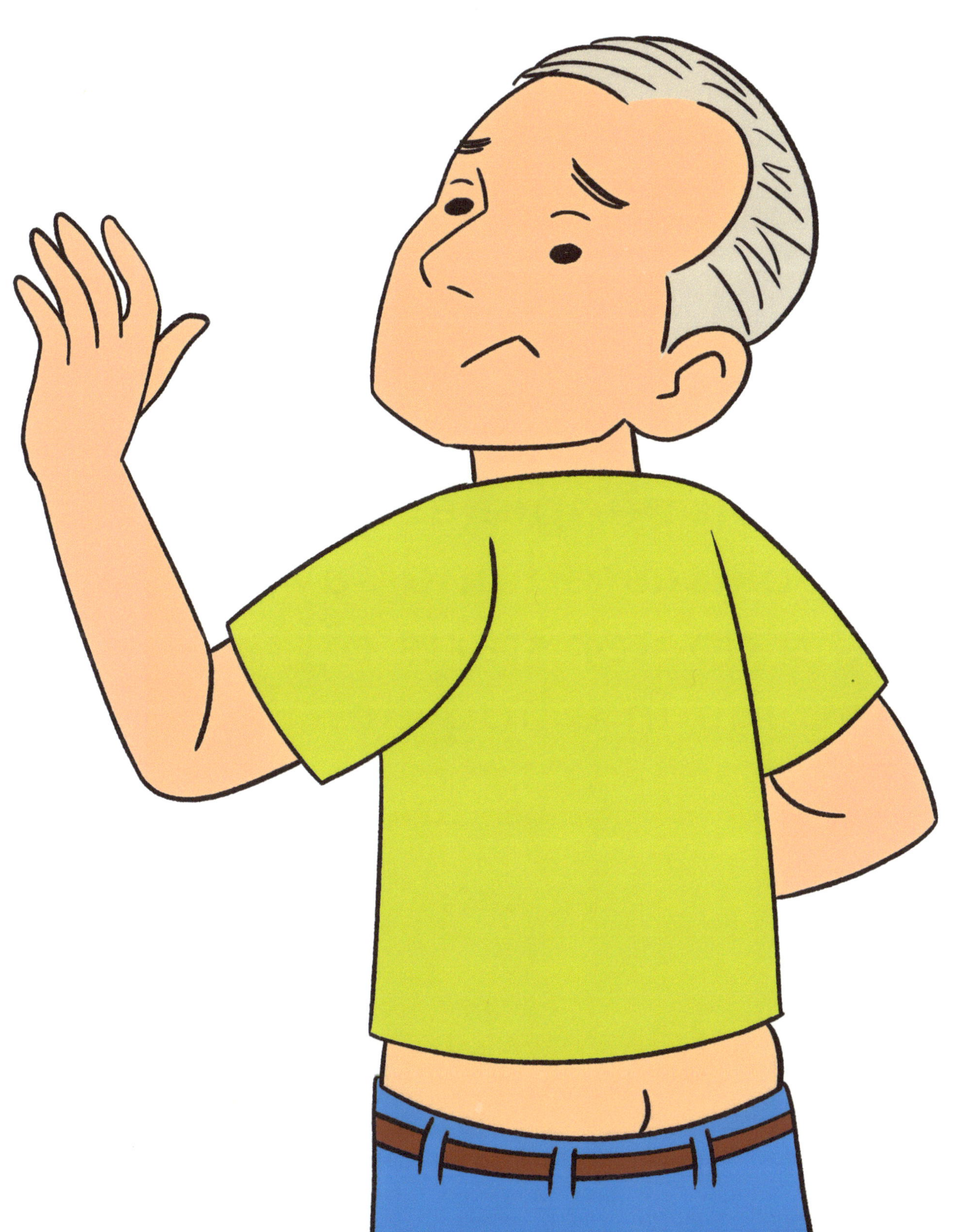

When I tell people about it,
They look scared and say "oh my."
Like the doctor starts off,
Putting me in a hog-tie.

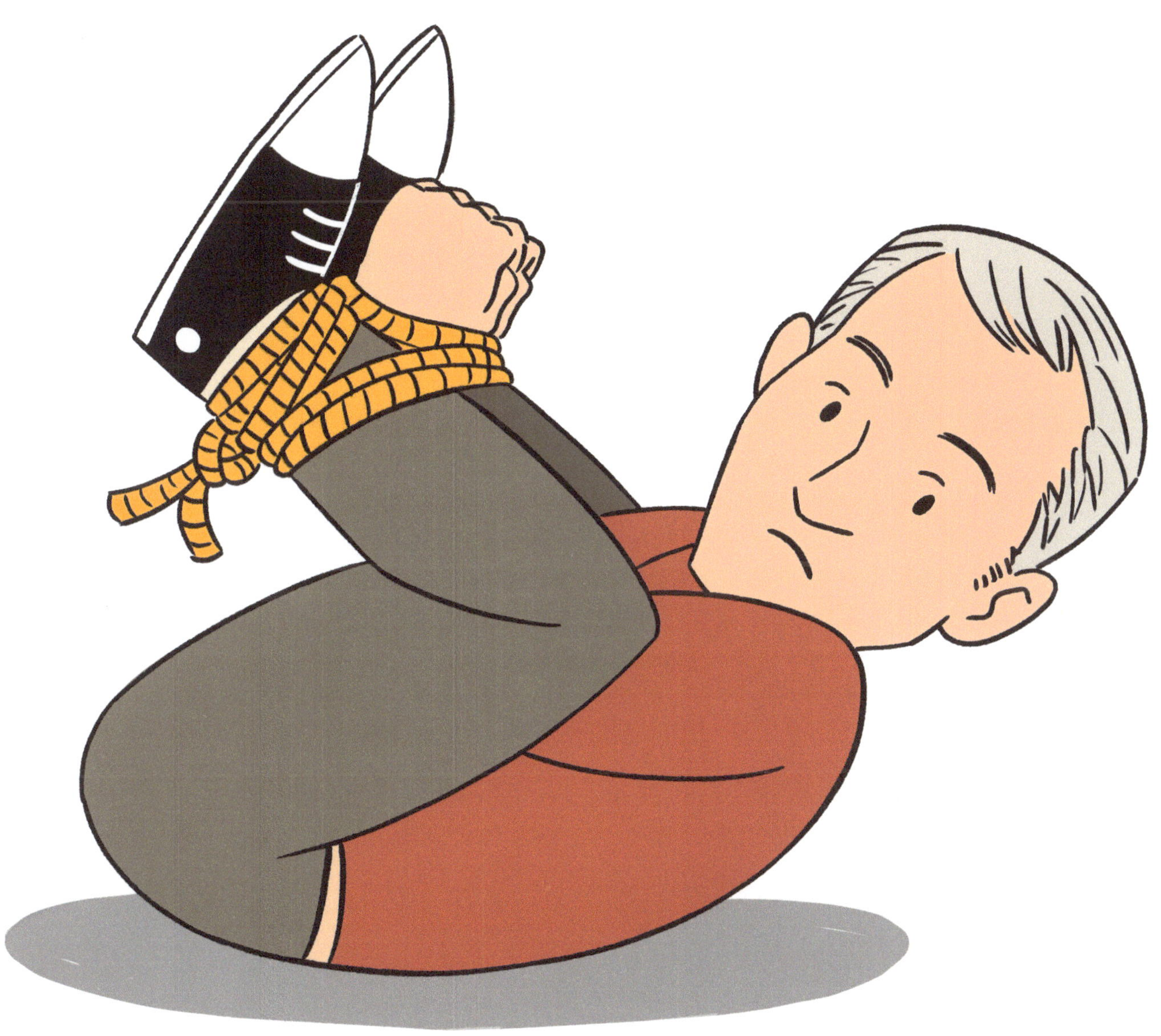

The laxative they gave me,
They said to "clean me out."
It was like my rear end
Became a water spout.

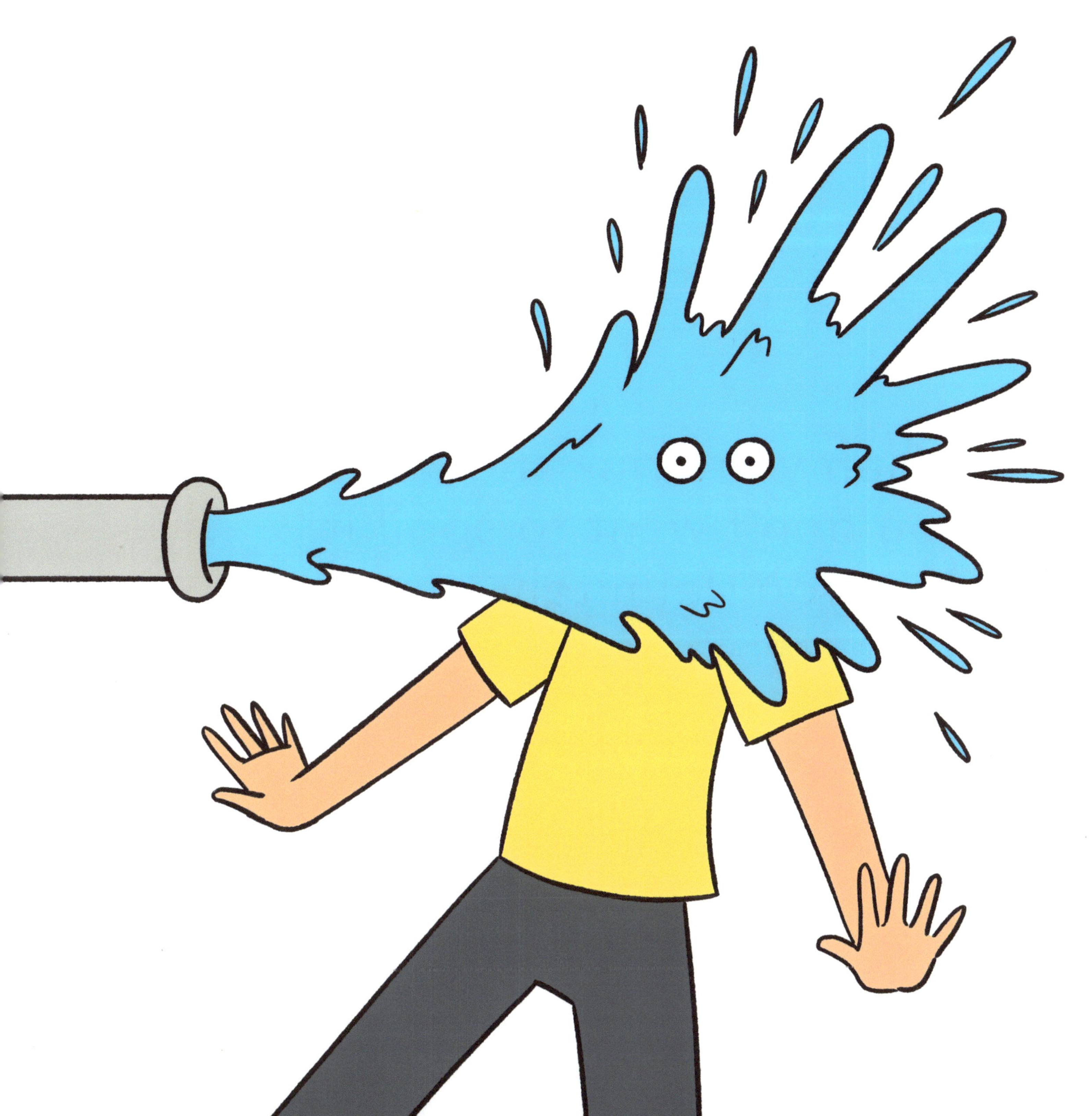

When you drink the laxative,
You don't want to spoil it.
And you definitely want to be near,
Your own favorite toilet.

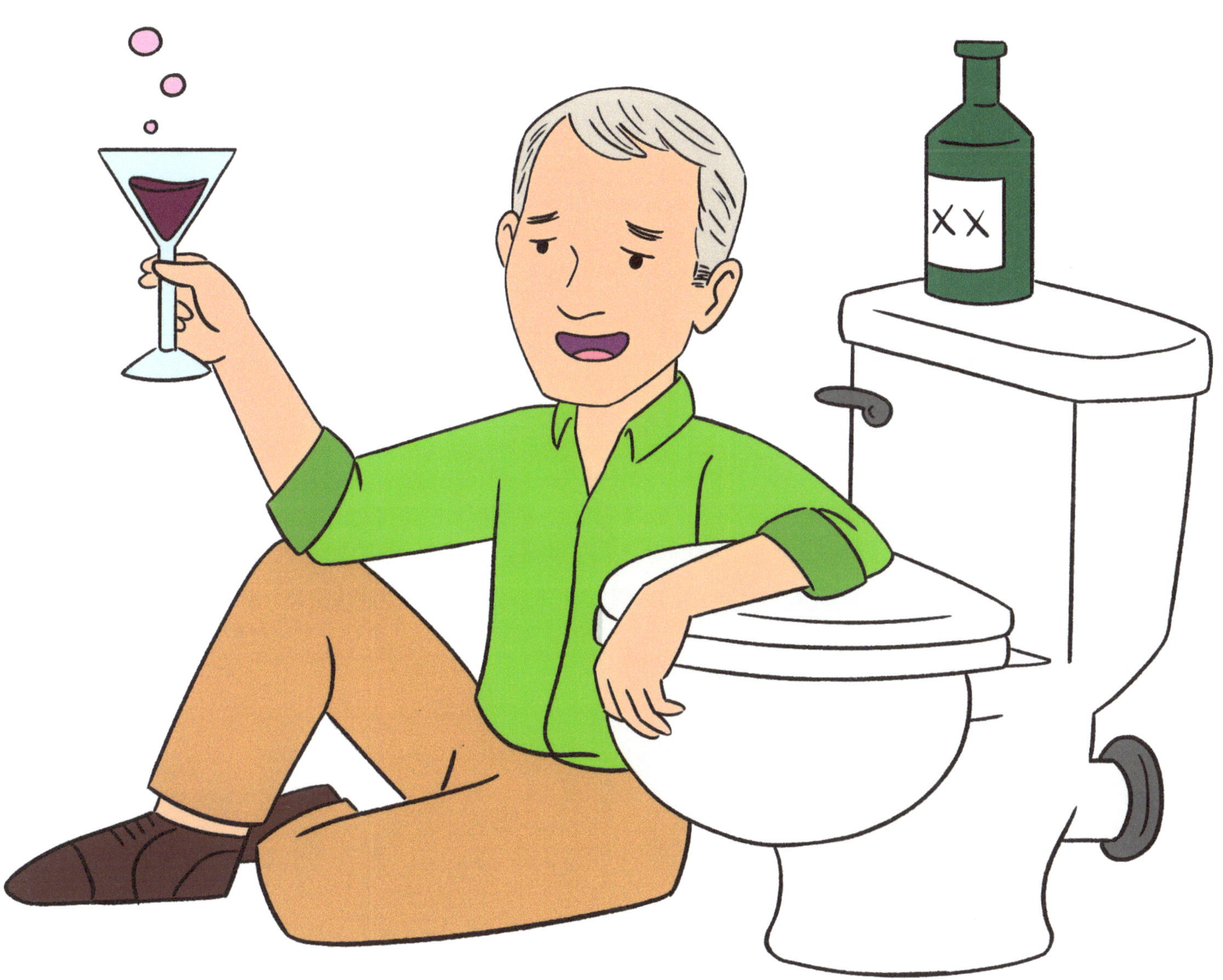

Yes I was a bit nervous,
And a bit horrified.
To have some doctor,
Fishing in my backside.

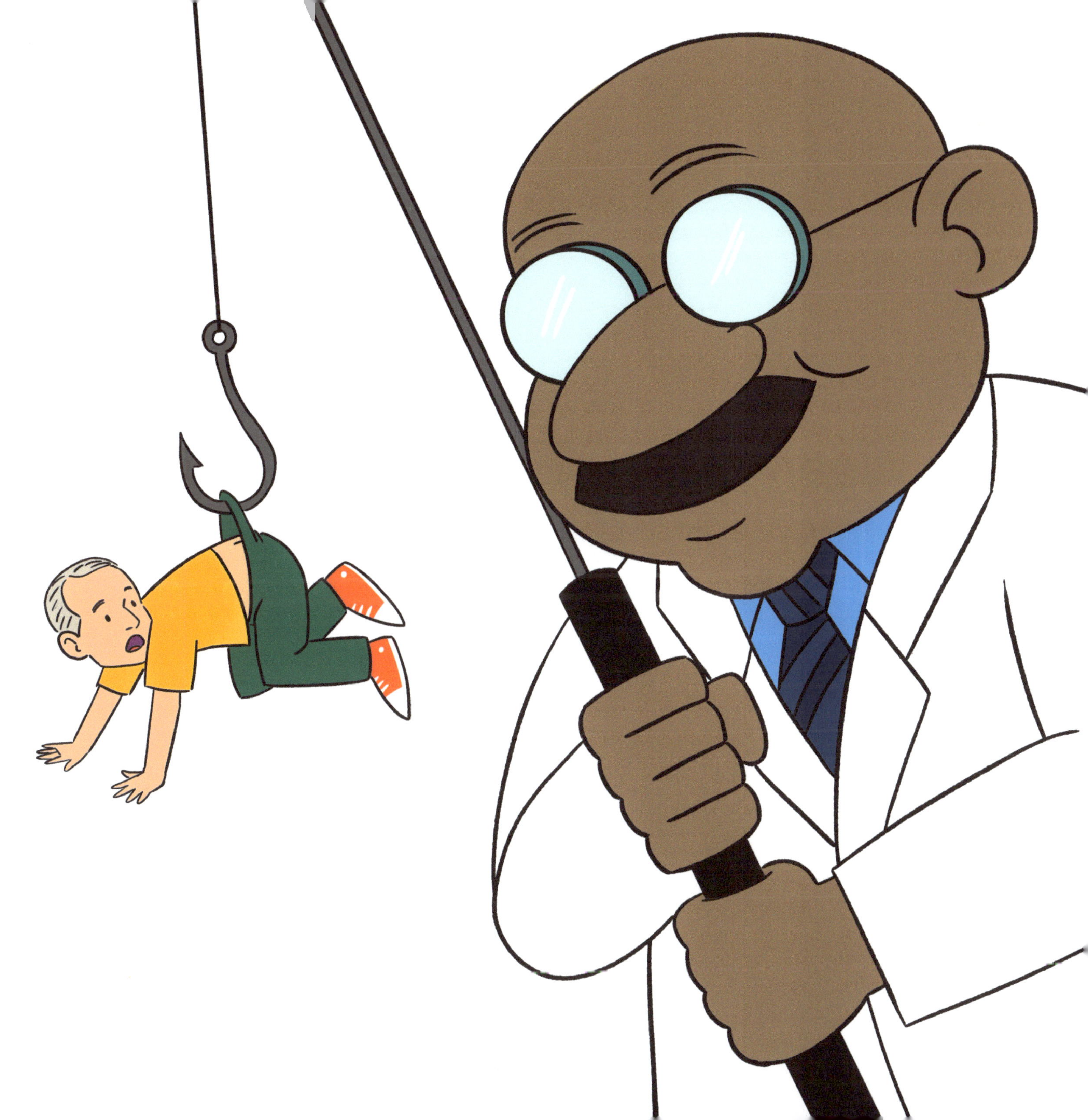

When going to the procedure,
I had feelings of misplacement.
Because I felt like I was going,
To some weirdo's basement.

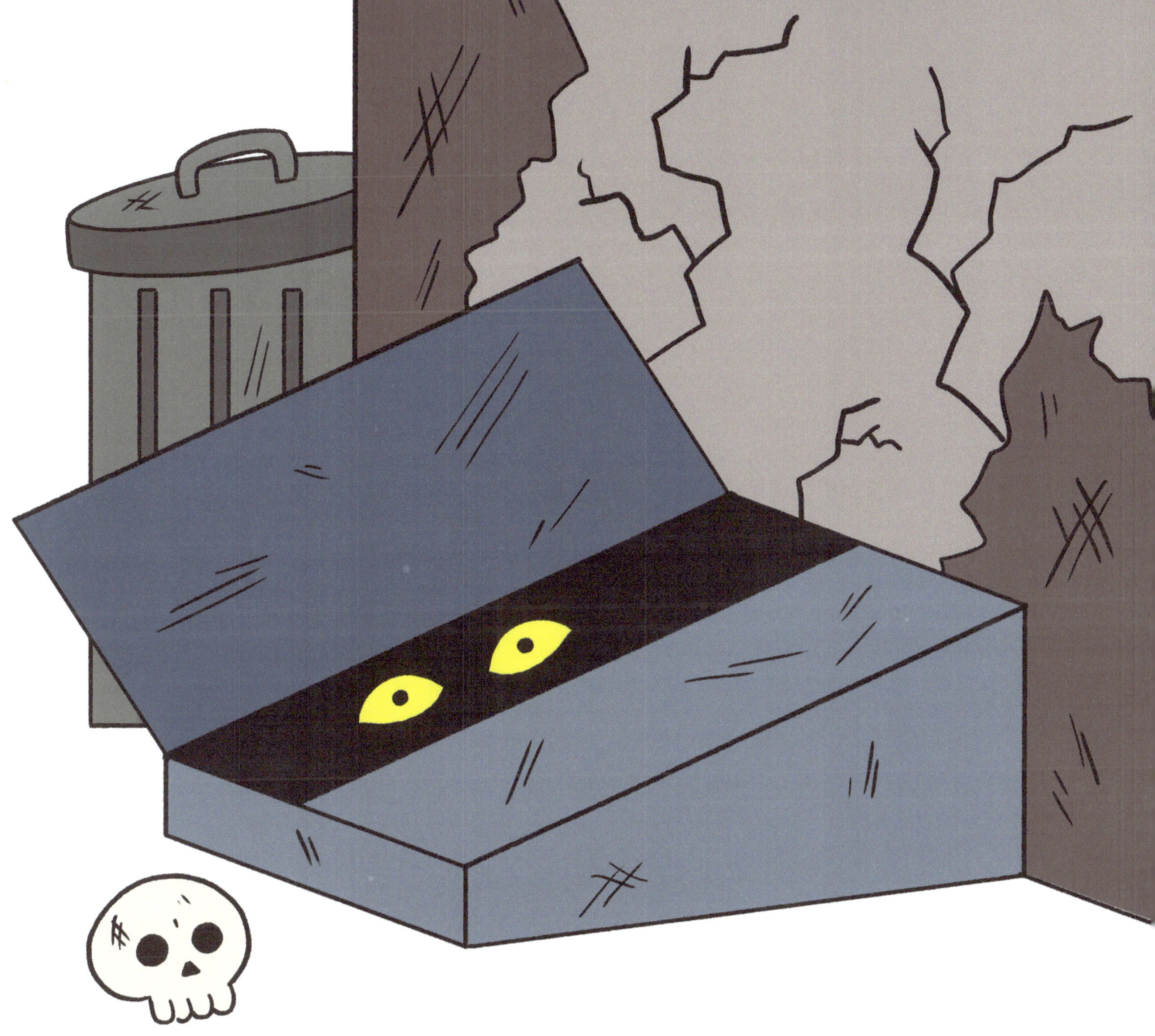

I gave them consent,
And I knew for what.
To get some photos
Of inside my butt.

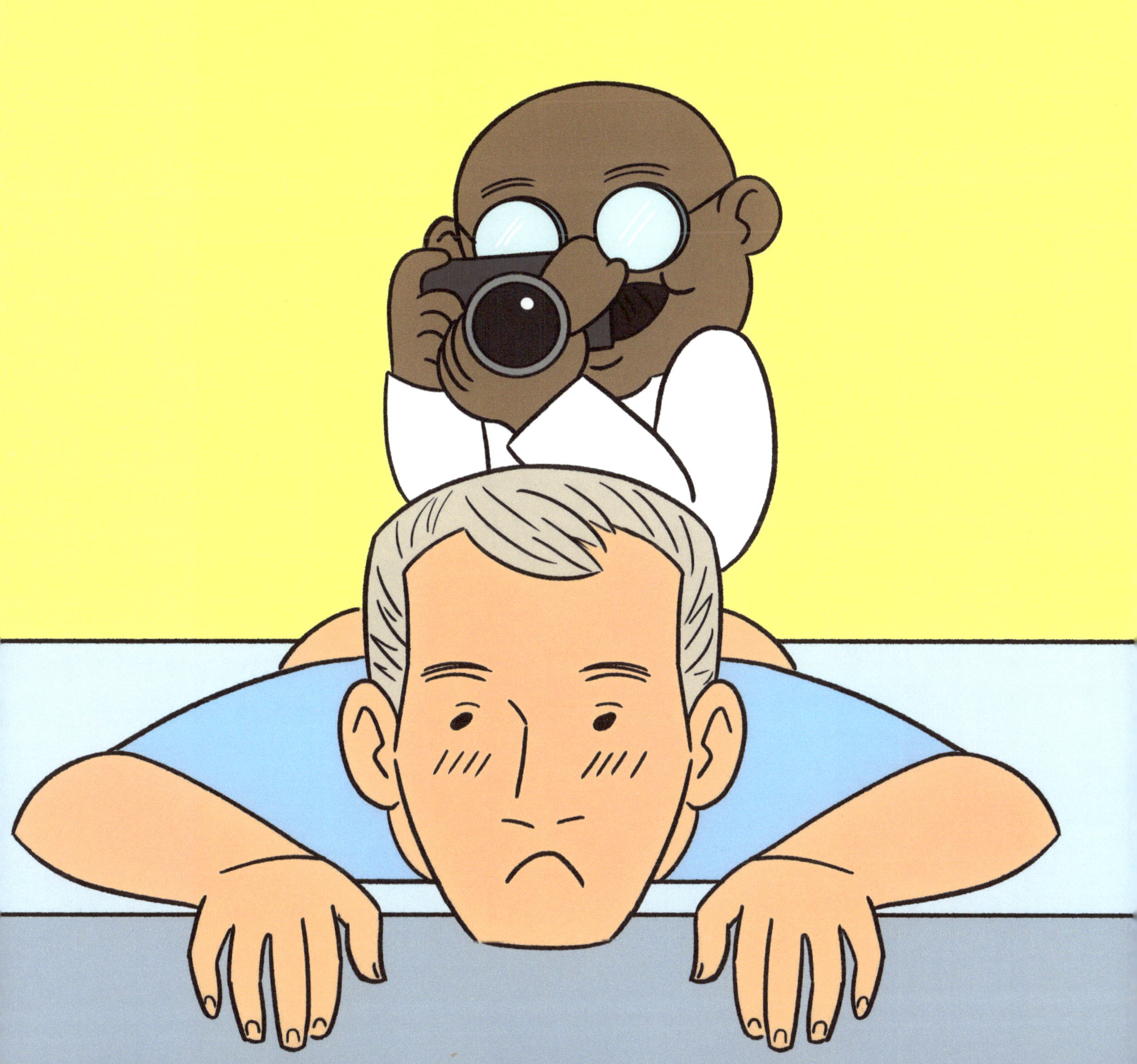

At the doctors office,
They greet you with a smile.
I can't believe these people,
Have chosen this lifestyle.

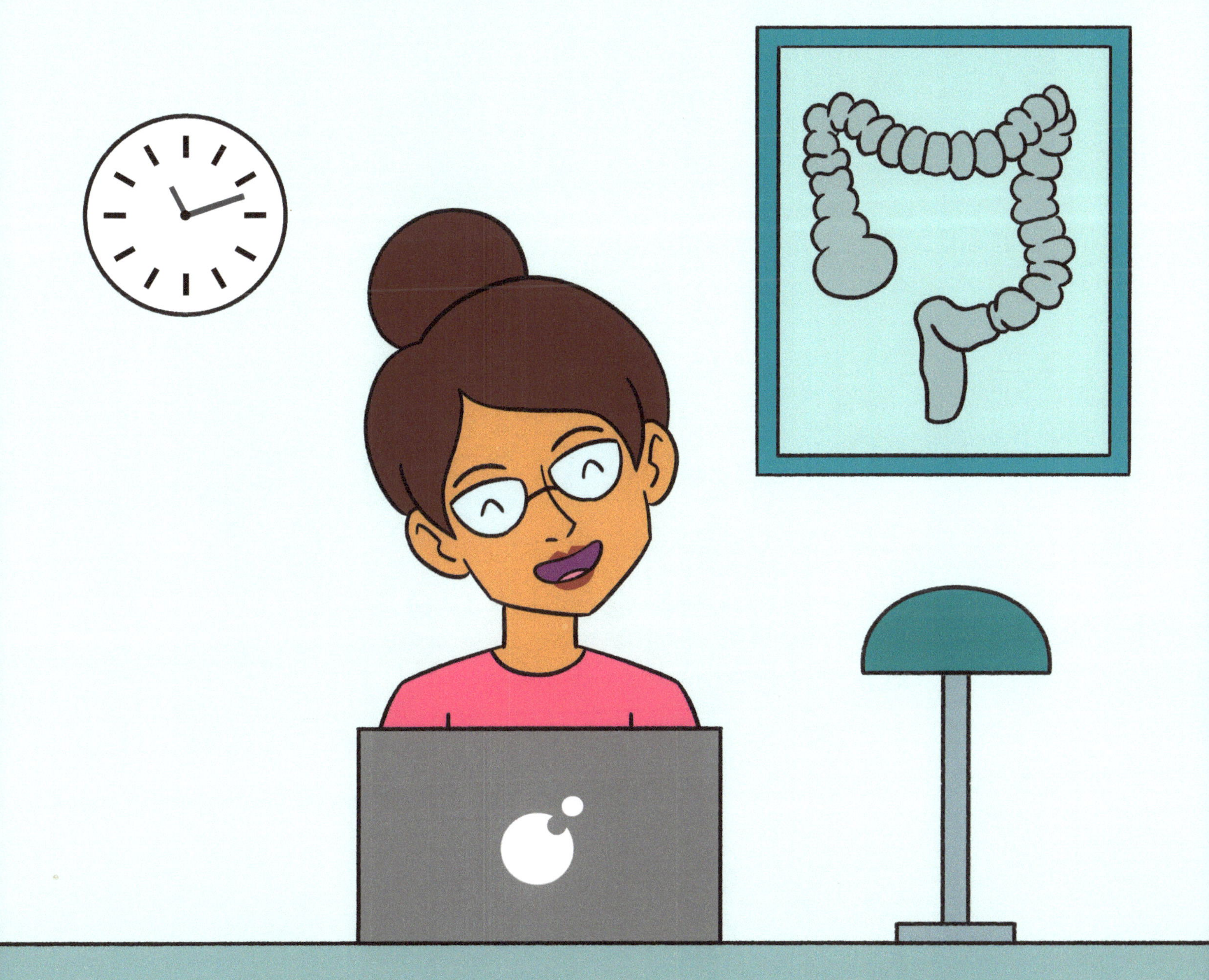

In the waiting room I sit,
And wonder why I'm here.
Fearing an early death,
Has strangers in my rear.

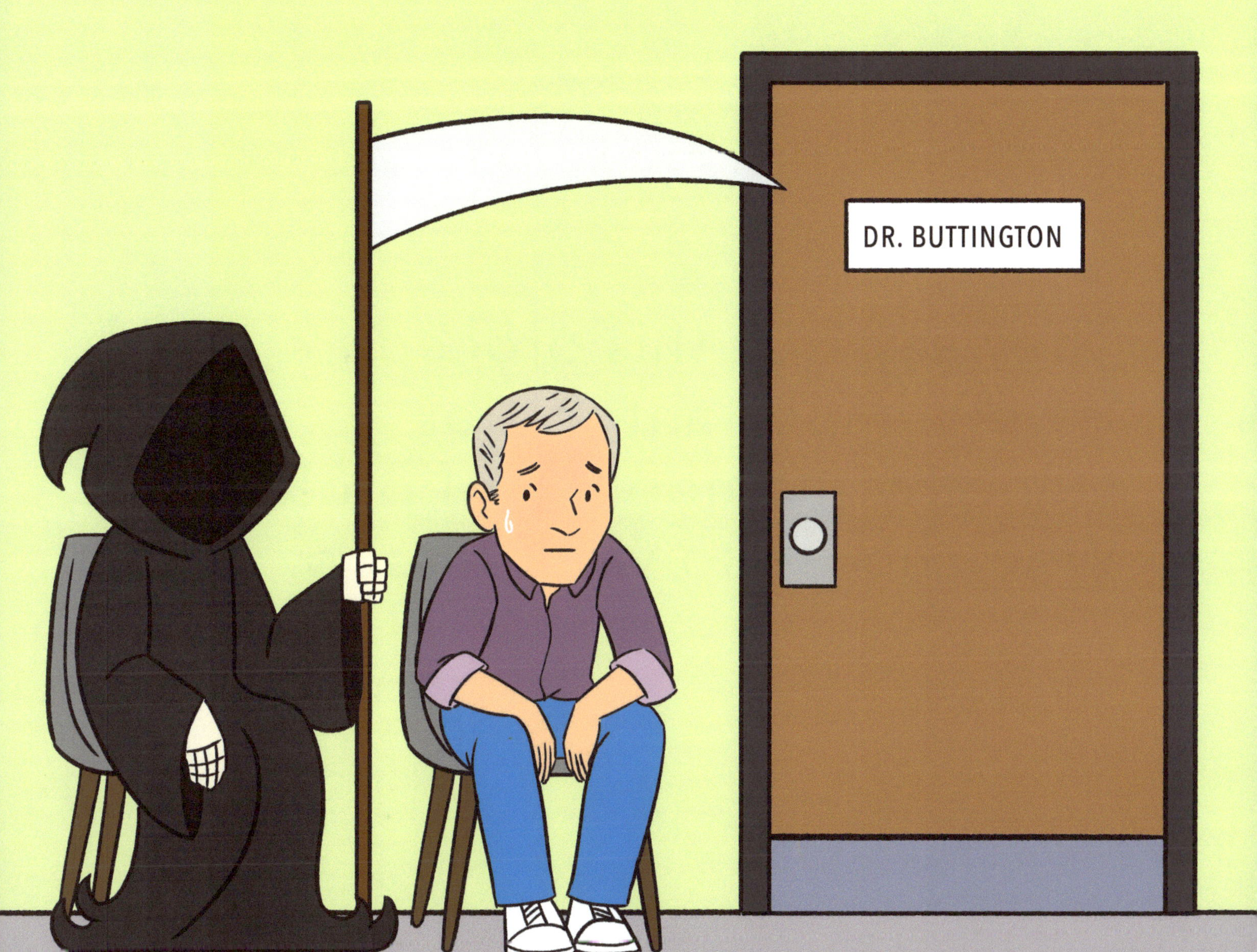
DR. BUTTINGTON

They say that this procedure,
Is very important to do.
Done by the noblest of professions,
Who choose to work in poo.

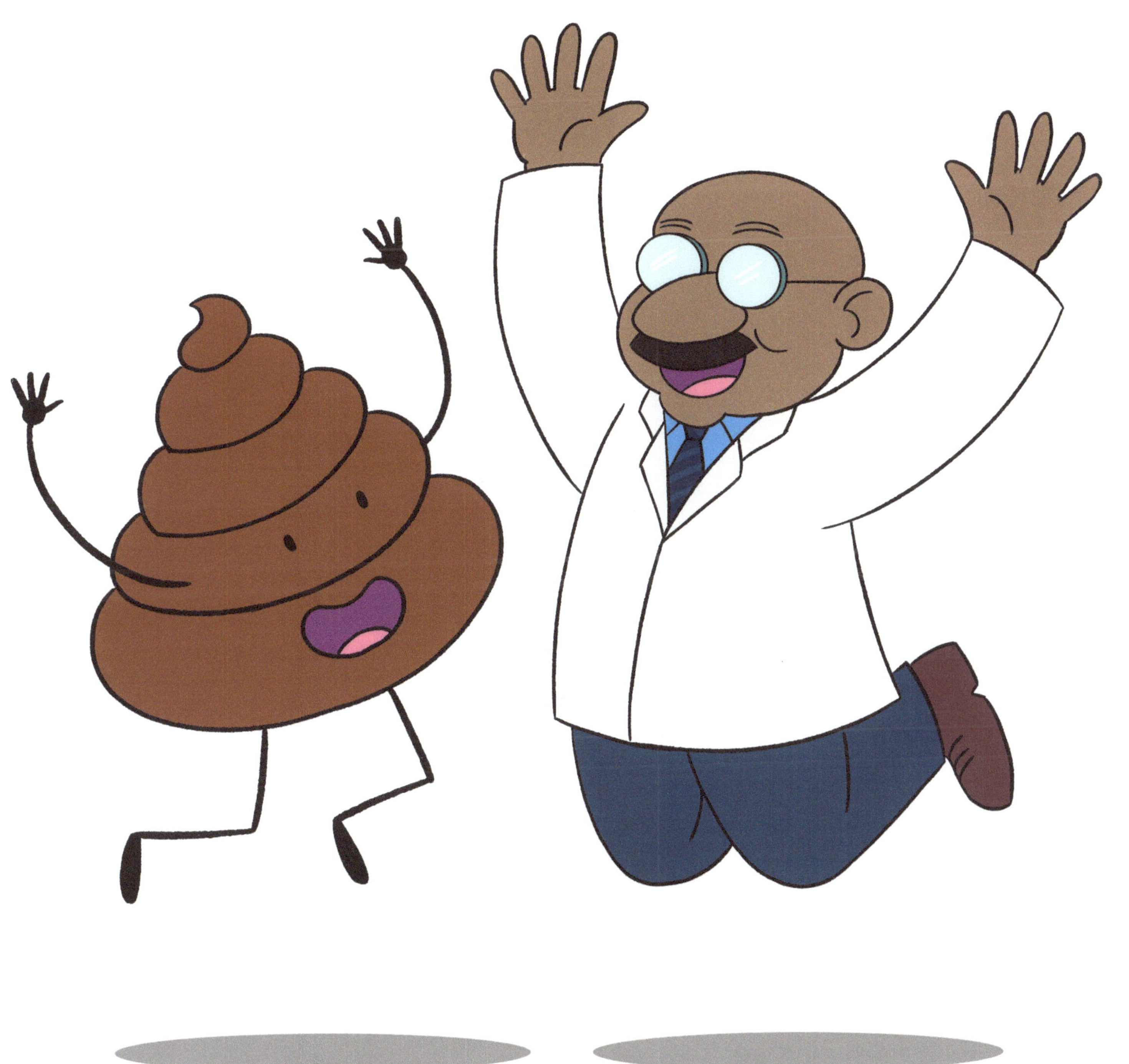

I fasted before the procedure,
And went into ketosis.
They went so far up my backside,
That it fixed my scoliosis.

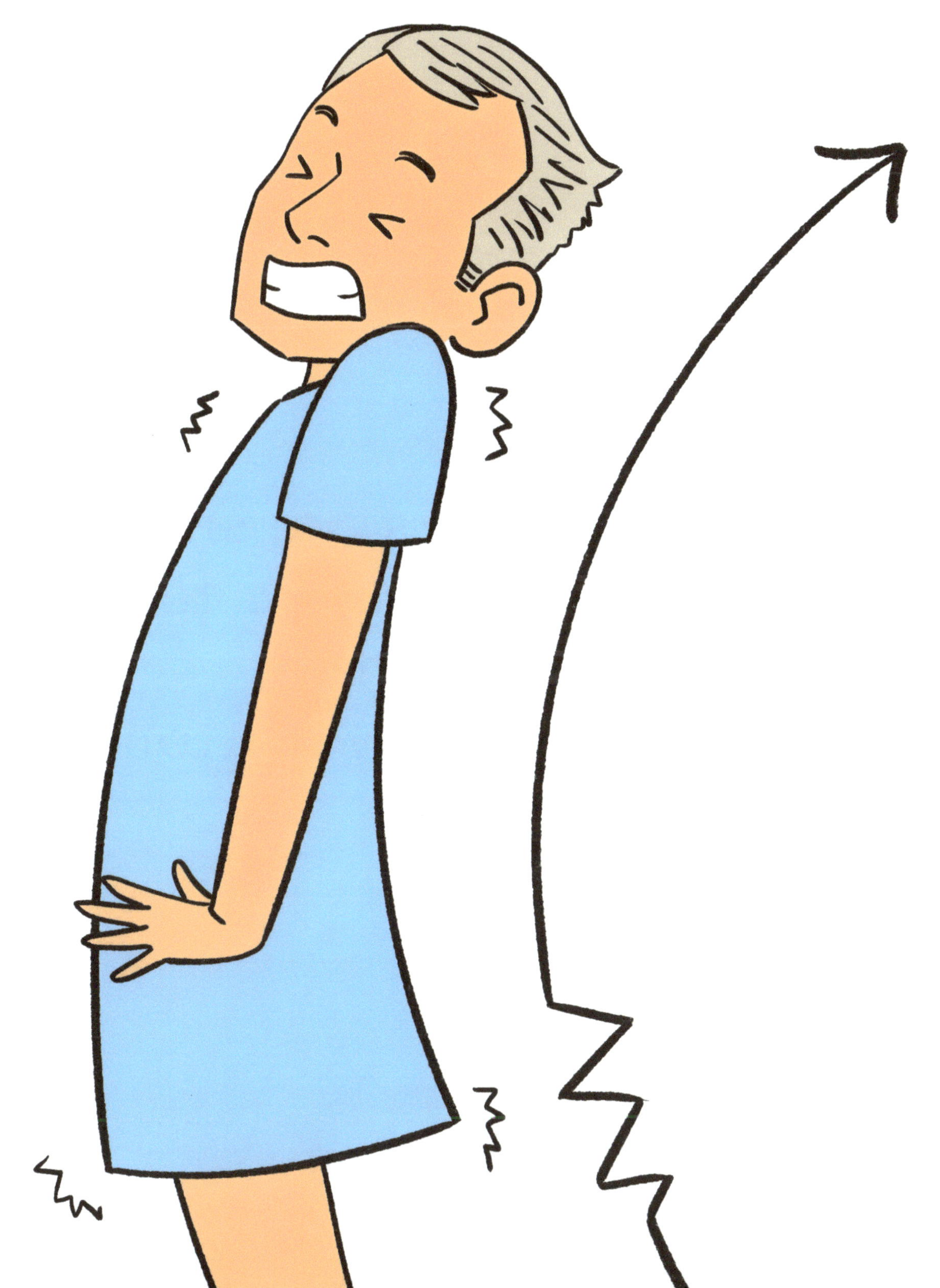

I know the doctors are smart,
But we don't know who taught 'em.
To be all professional,
When looking at my bottom.

HOW TO EXPLORE
THE HUMAN REAR
FOR MORONS

It is true that we need them,
And yes they do good work.
I just hope after today,
I'm still able to twerk.

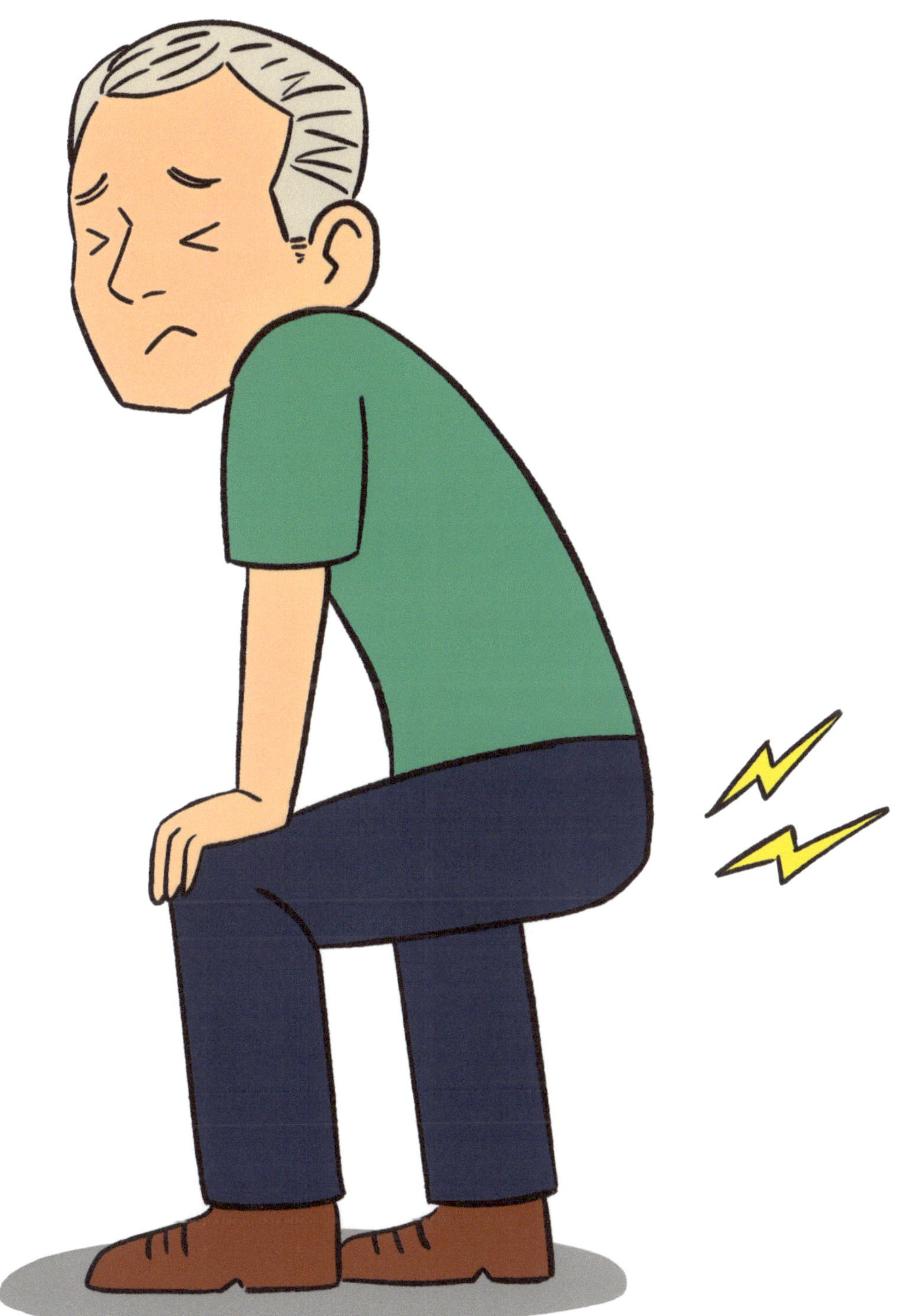

The procedure is done.
My head is still buzzin.
It oddly reminds me,
Of time with my cousin.

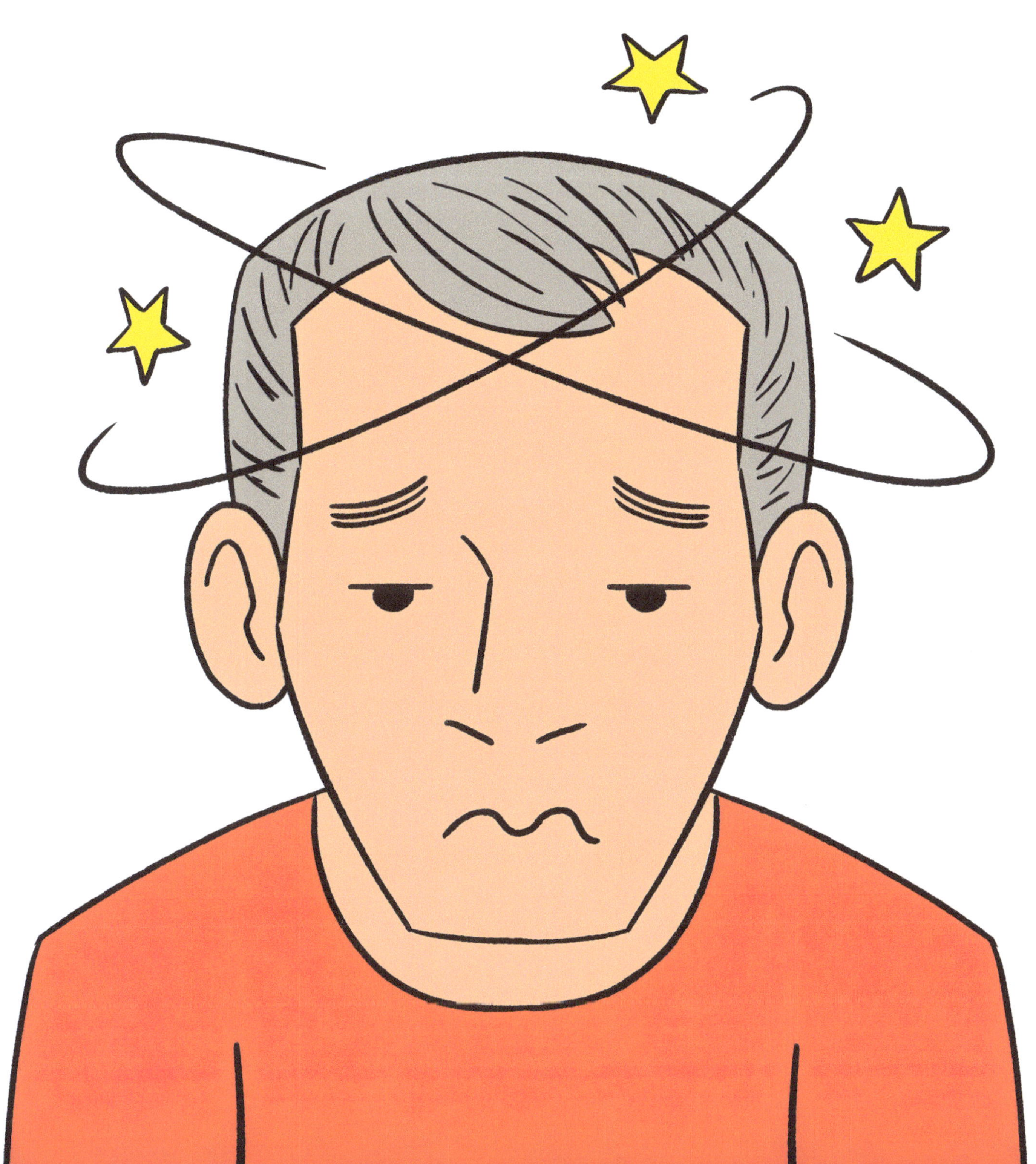

My wife drove me home,
Which was kinda lame.
But it wasn't the first time,
She saw my walk of shame.

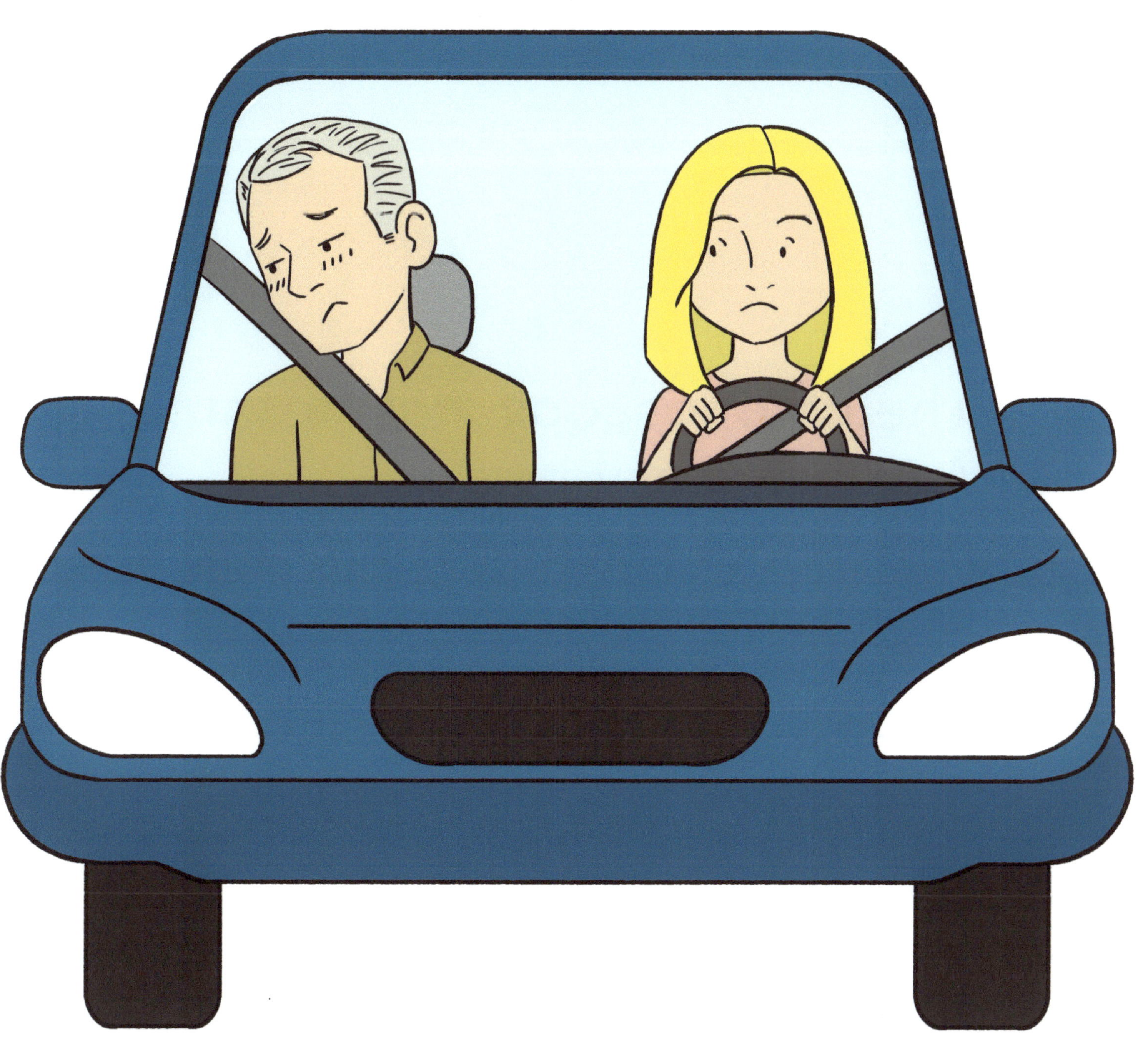

The colonoscopy was nothing,
And was easy to do.
It was like playing a game,
Of adult peek-a-boo.

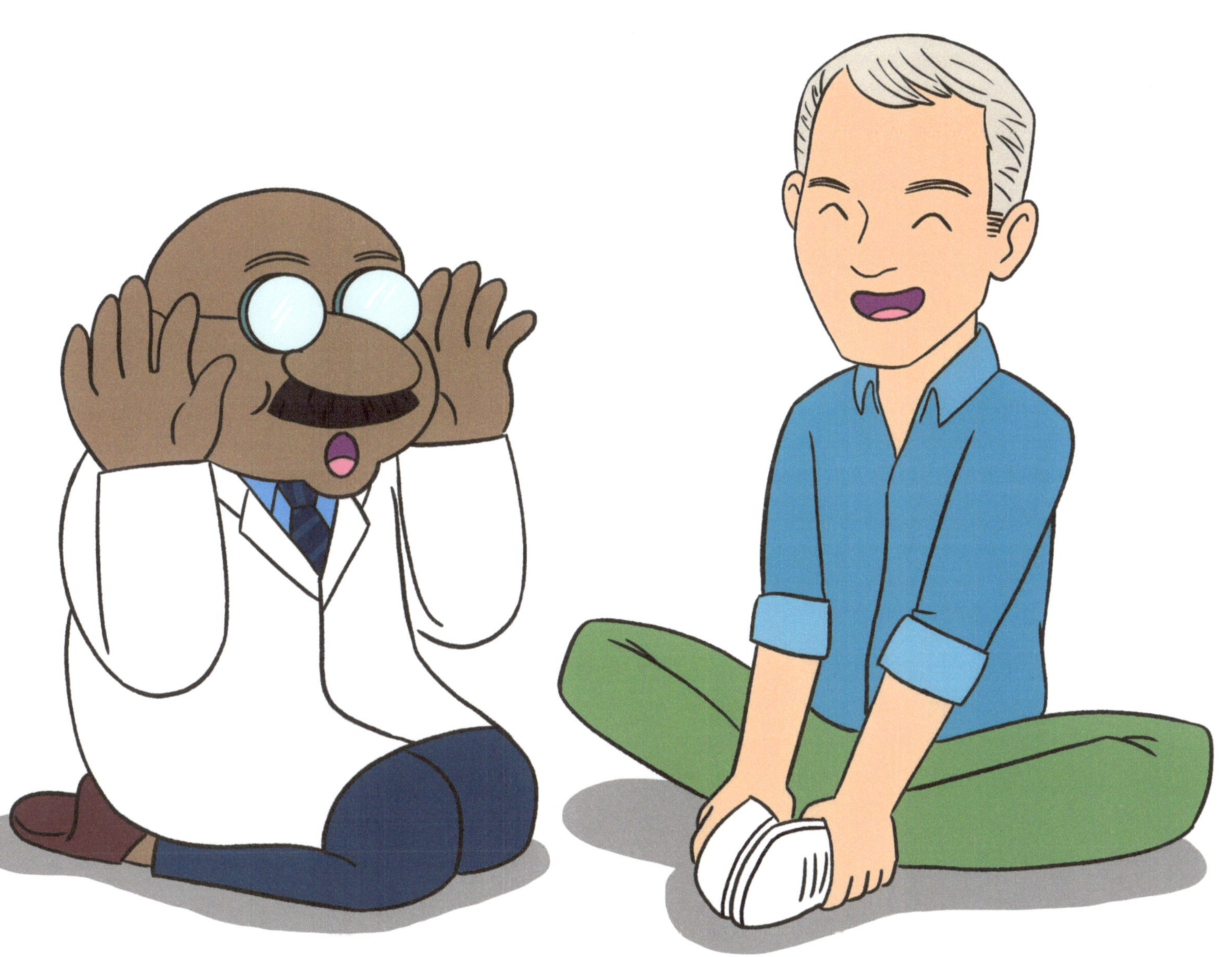

I am glad this is over,
And I was excited to leave.
I just hope my wife,
Likes my new boyfriend Steve.

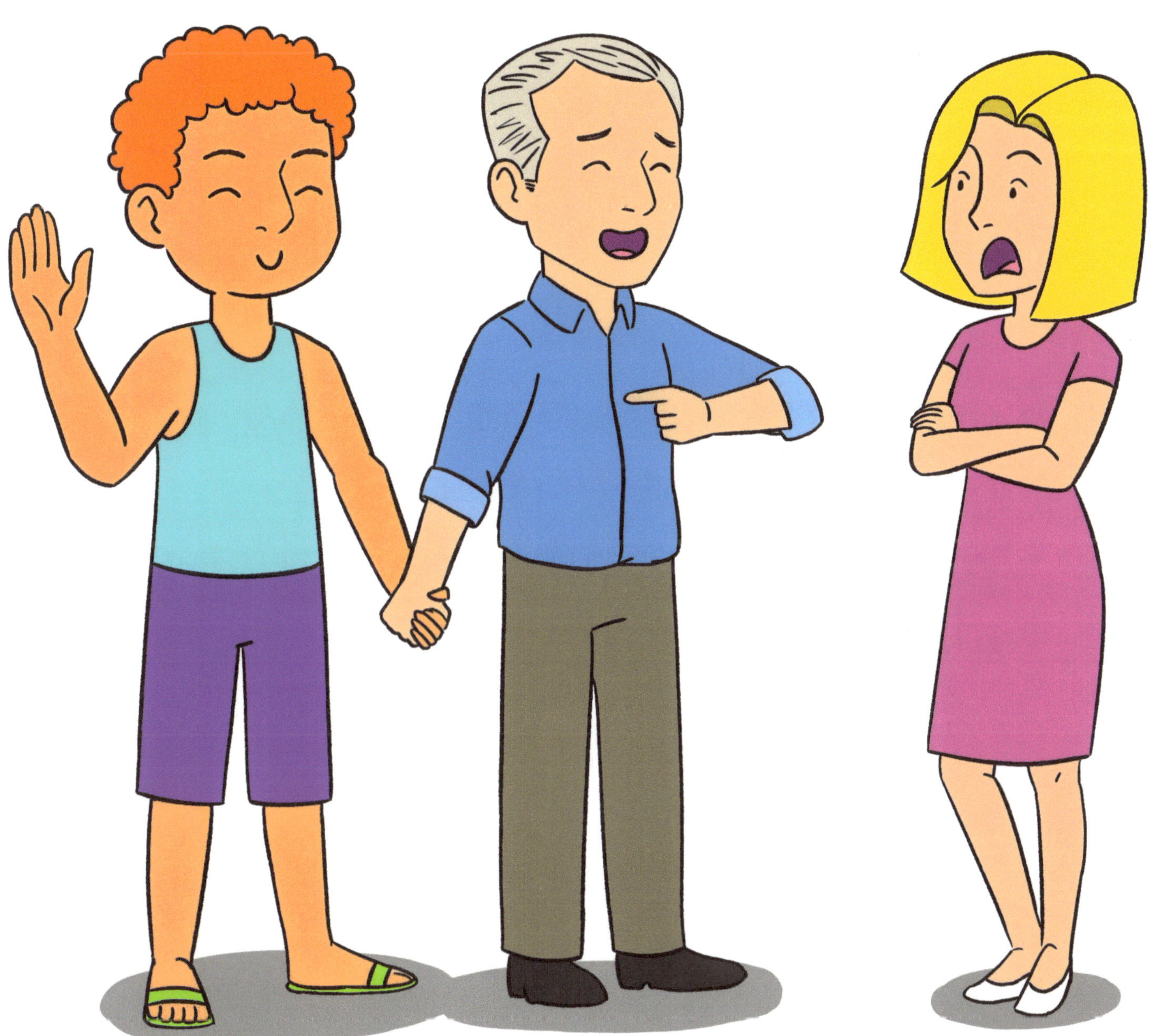

The worst part of the day,
Was before it took place.
I was so scared and confused,
I almost brought mace.

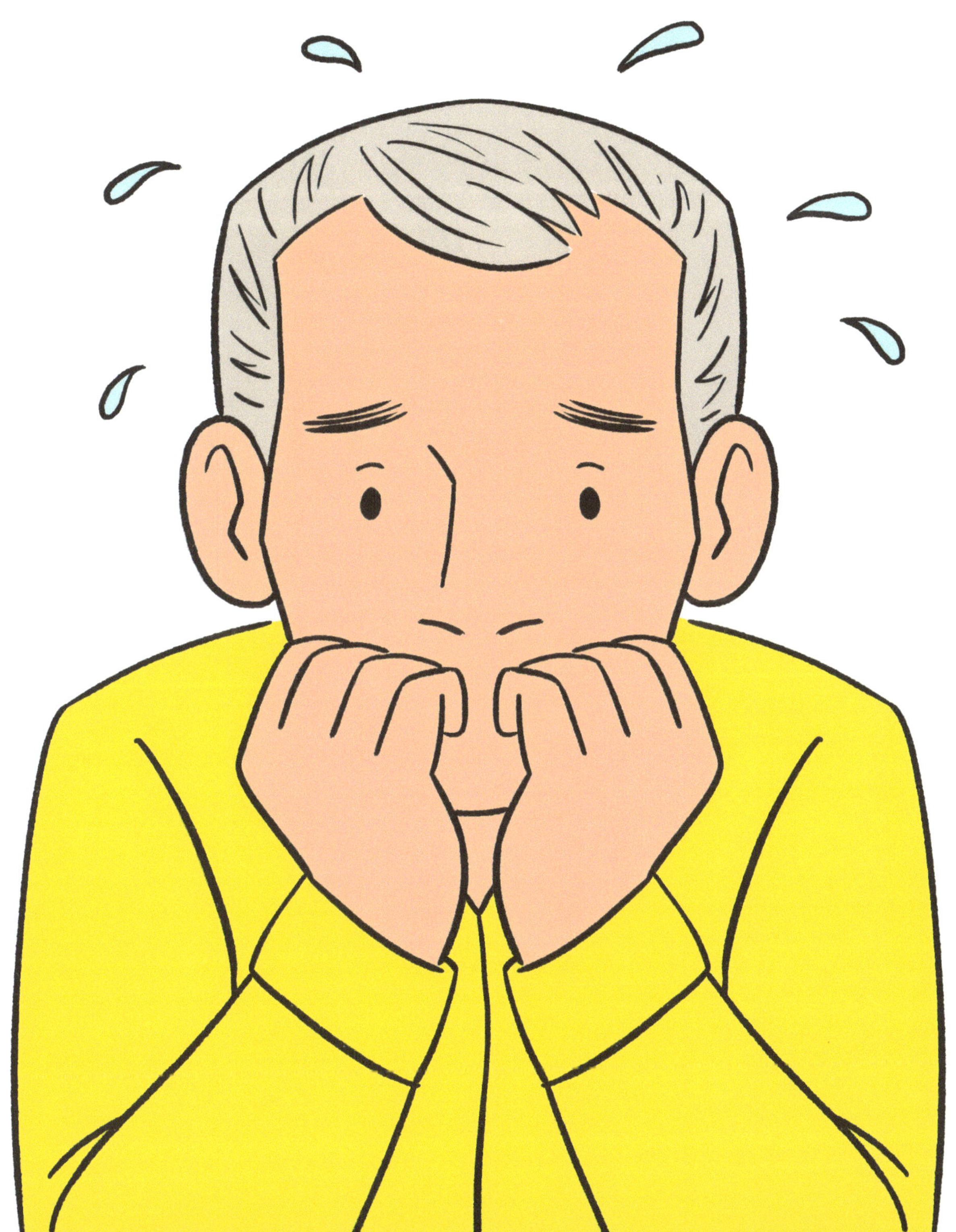

If you are debating about
this procedure,
Then here is your answer:
Would you rather have this exam,
Or end up with cancer?

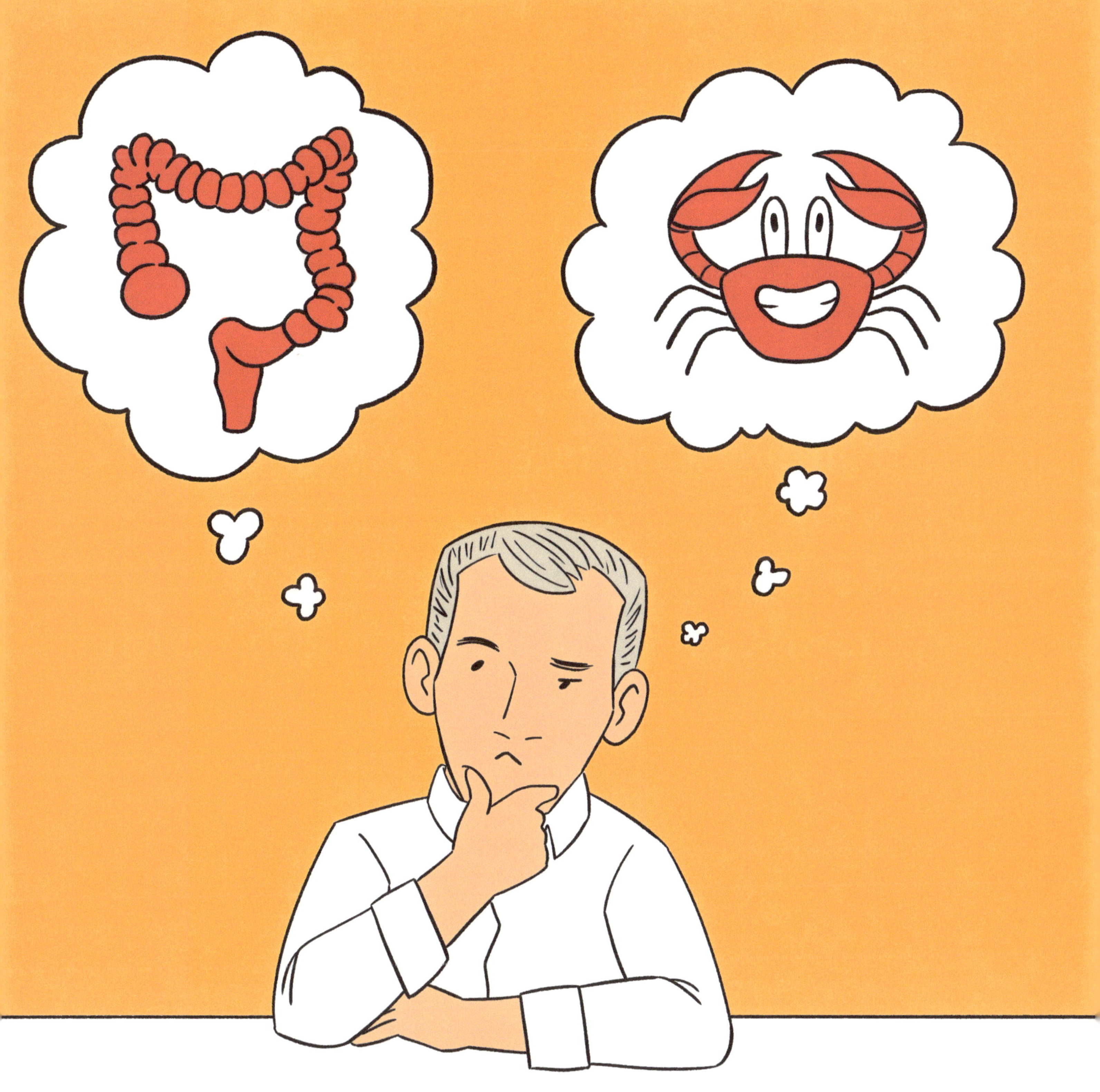

I believe this is an easy choice,
If you want to avoid getting ill.
Plus I found this colonoscopy
Was more like a Netflix and chill.

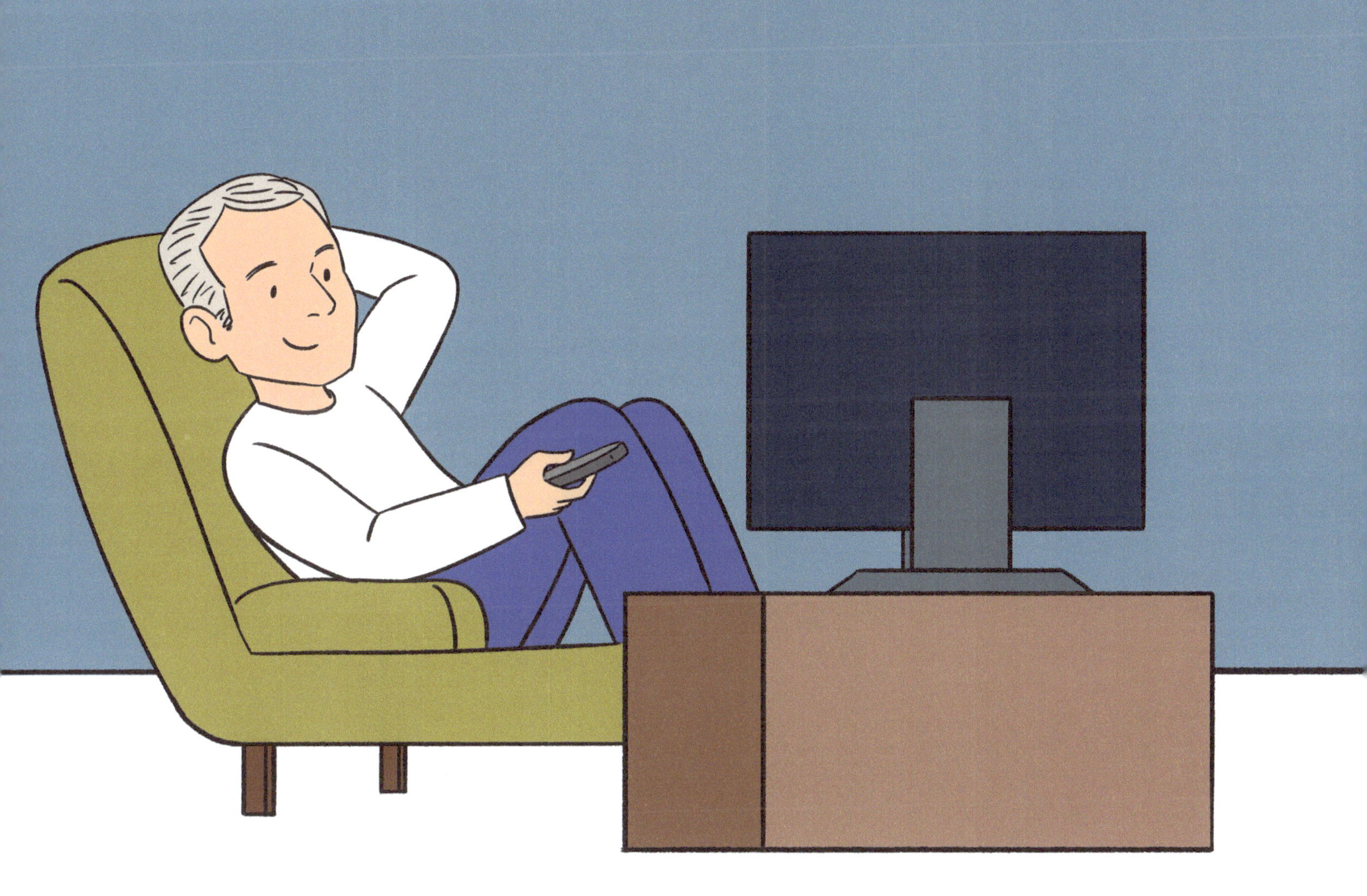

Stupid is as stupid does,
So says Forrest Gump.
But nothing is more stupider,
Than not checking out your rump.

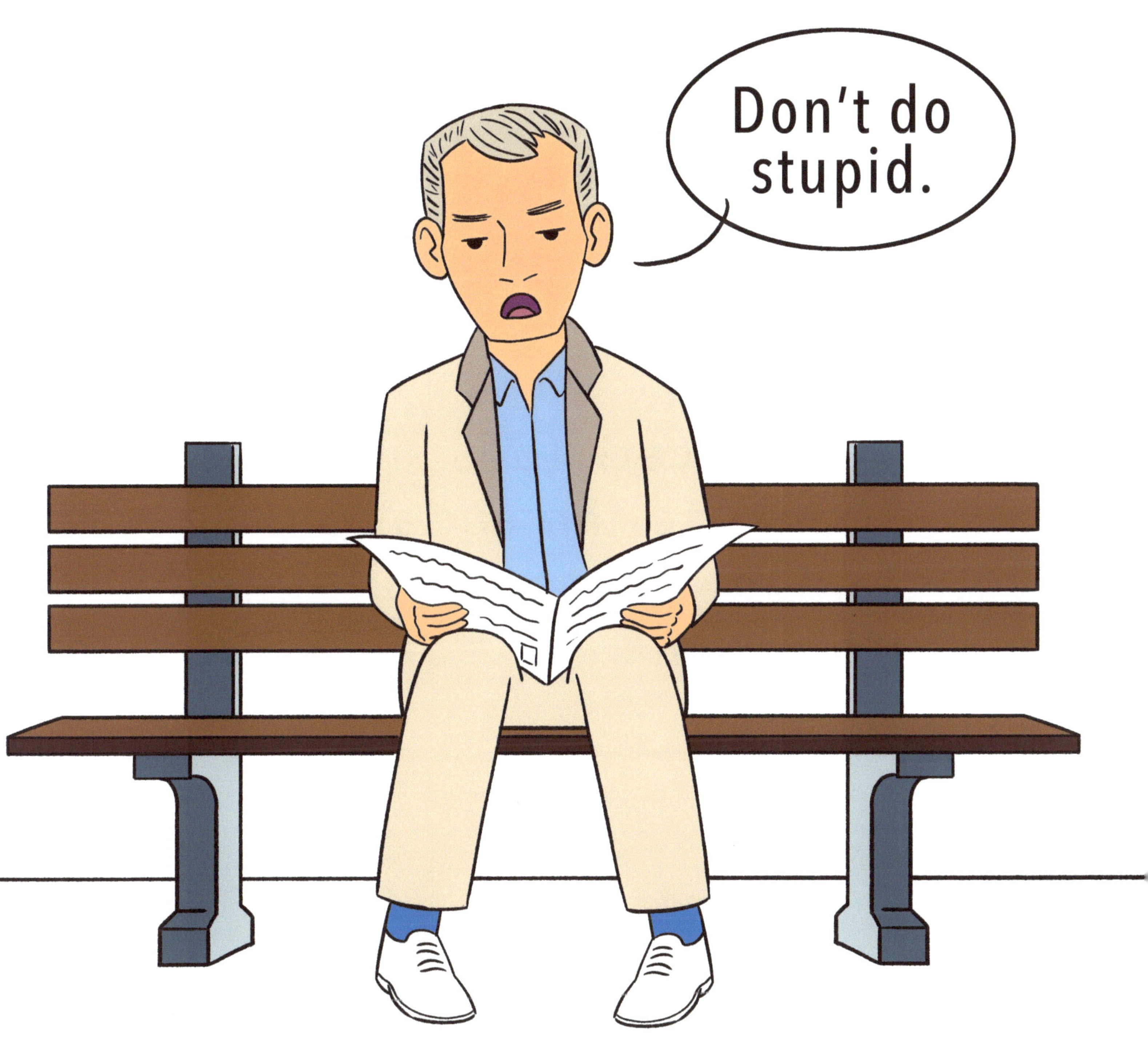
Don't do
stupid.

The procedure is simple,
Thanks to the sedation.
And my doctor was friendly,
He's in the right occupation.

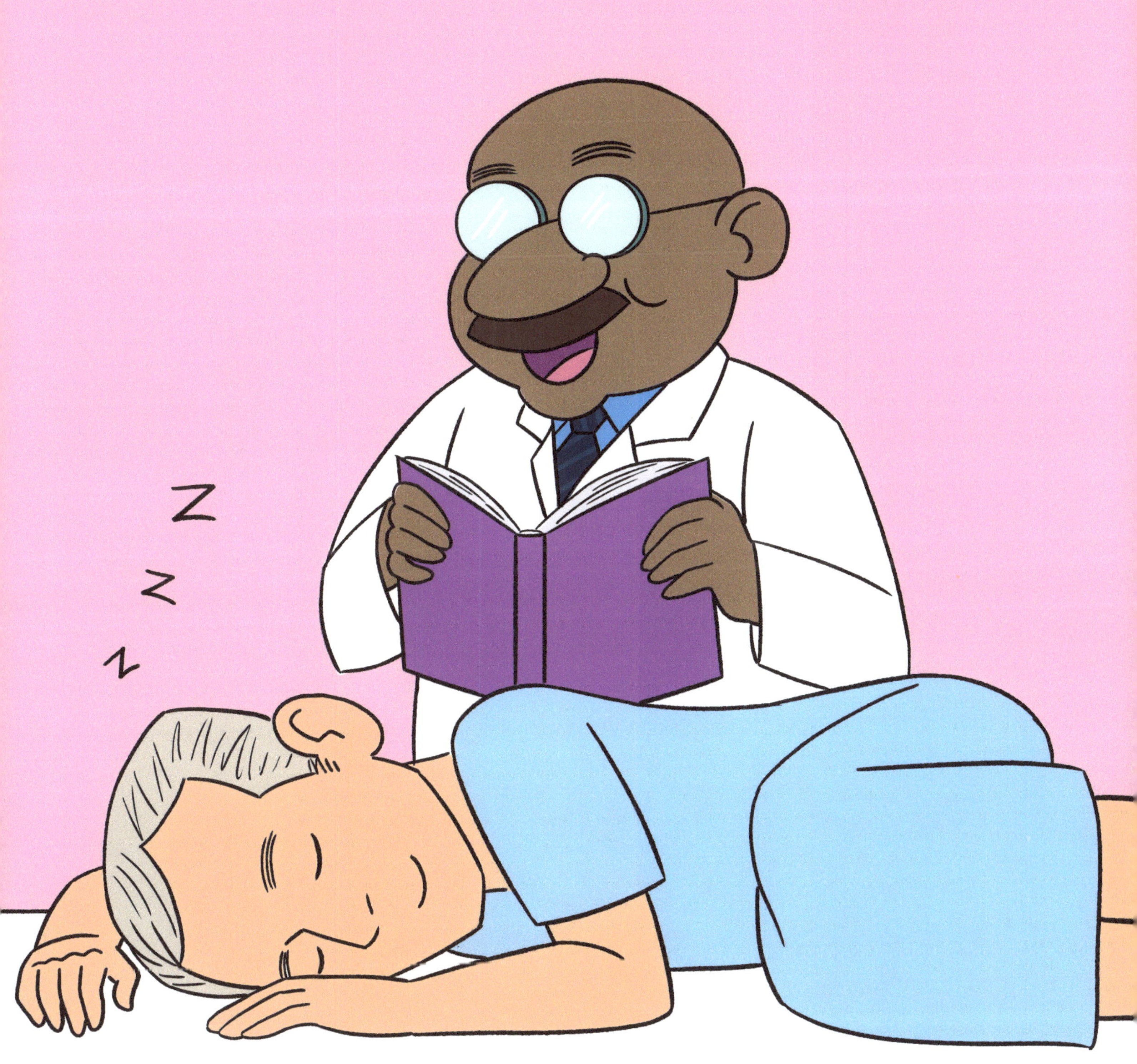

A colonoscopy is not as bad,
As my annual appointment.
Where the doctor uses one finger,
And very little ointment.

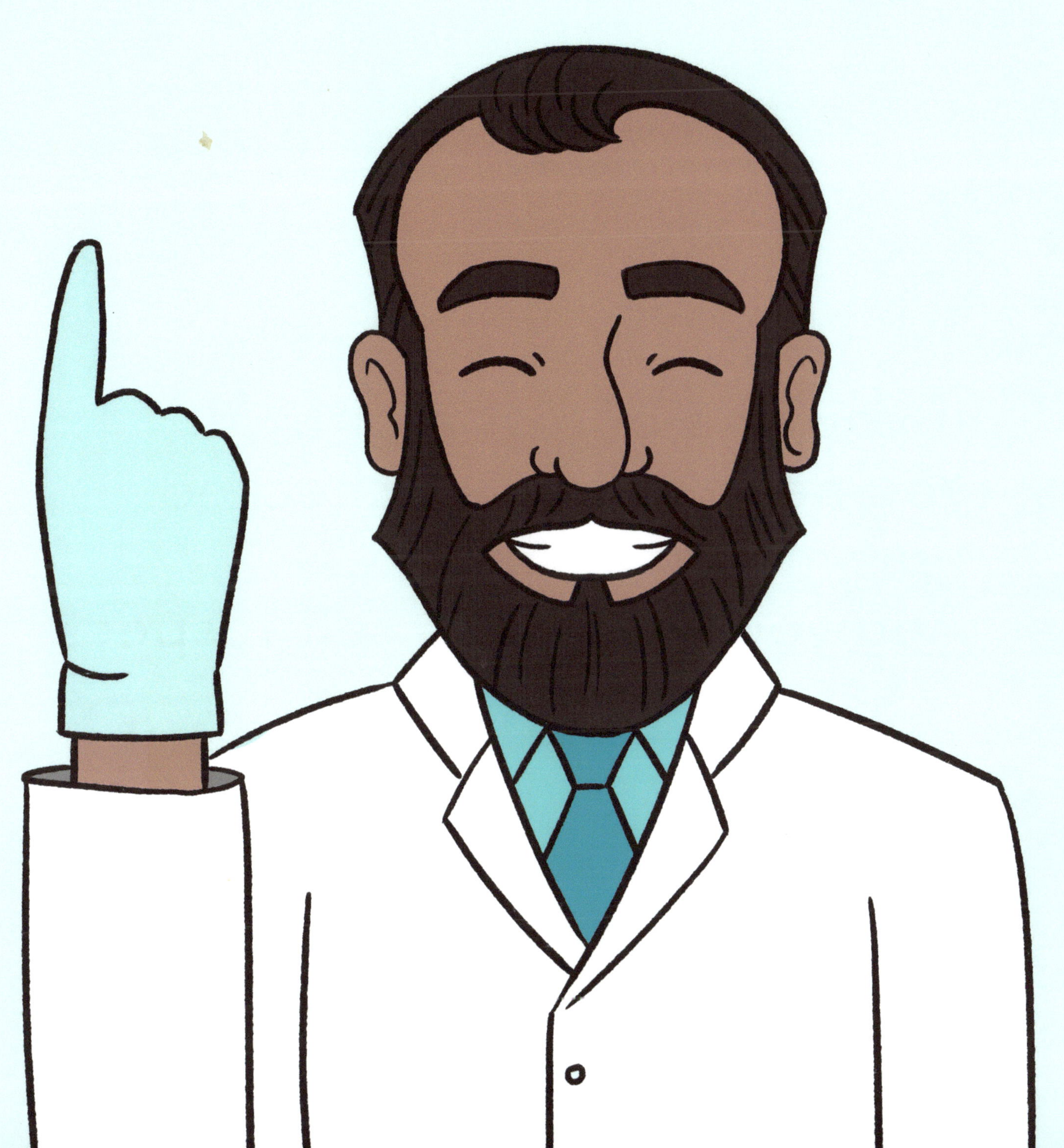

If you're a boy or a girl,
You need to go get checked.
I promise it's worth it,
And you won't lose self-respect.

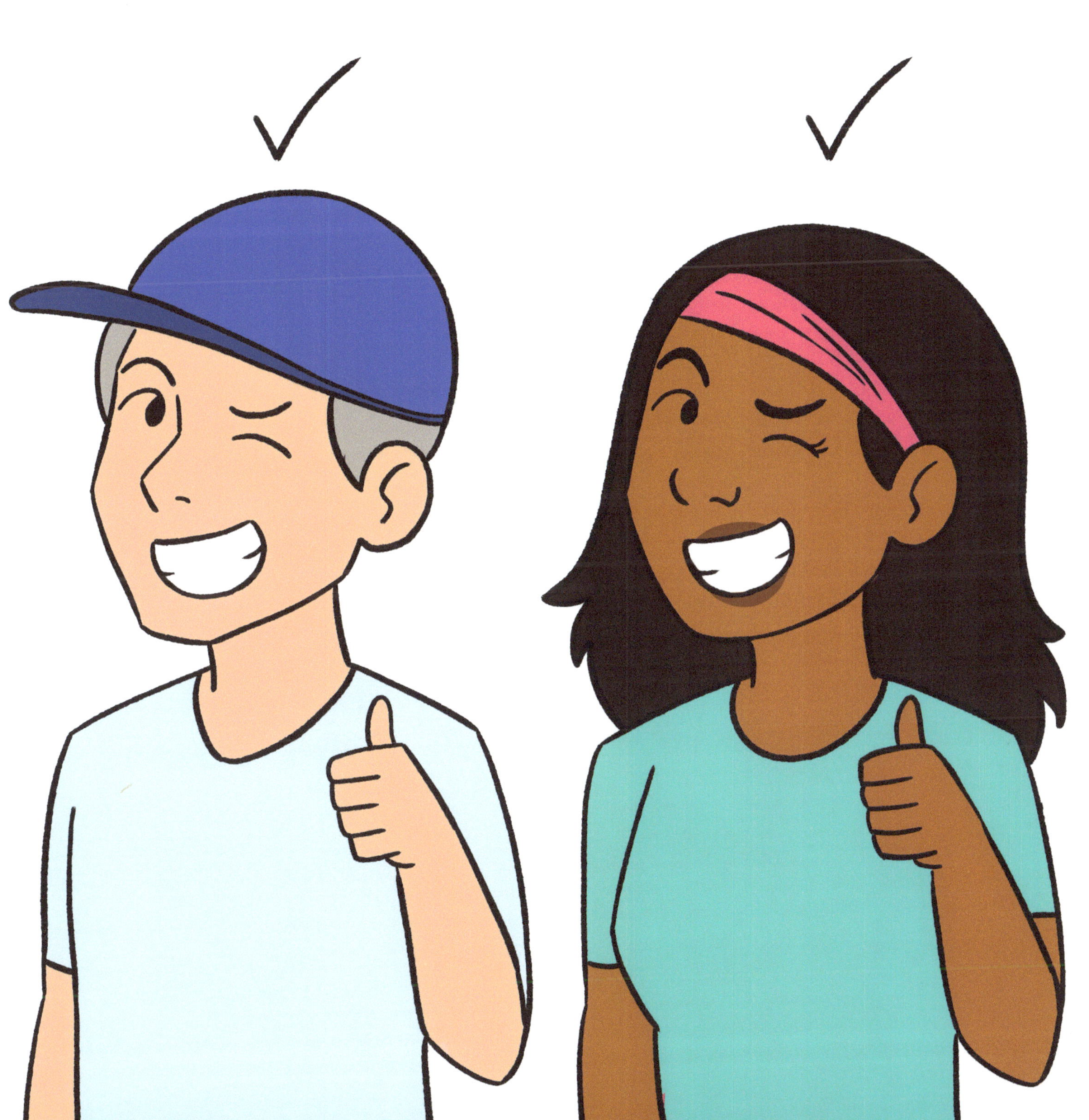

Getting checked out is smart,
And it will help to please ya.
You will not remember it,
It's like you got amnesia.

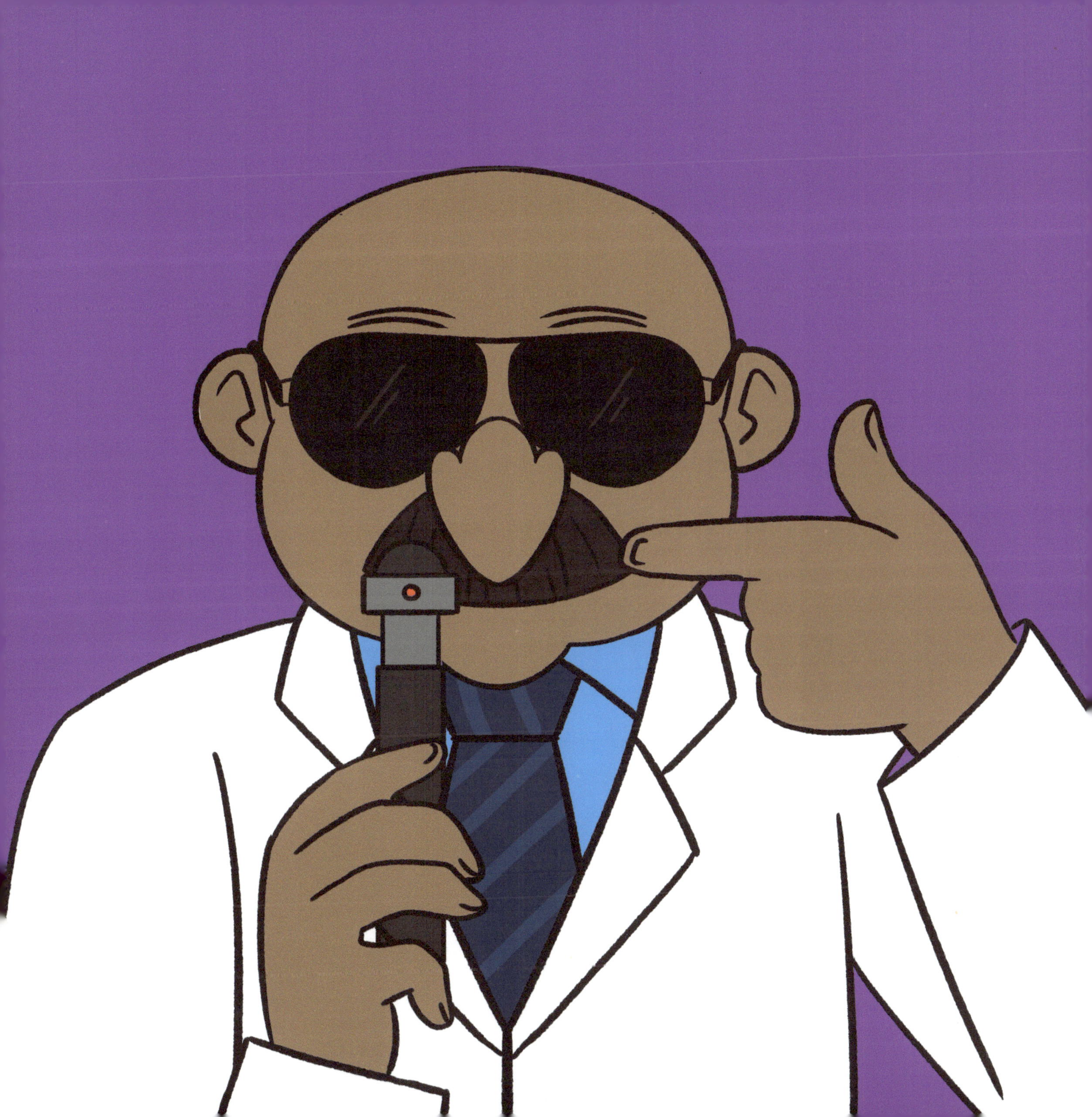

So call up your doctor,
And fill out the form.
Then brace yourself
For quite the poop-storm.

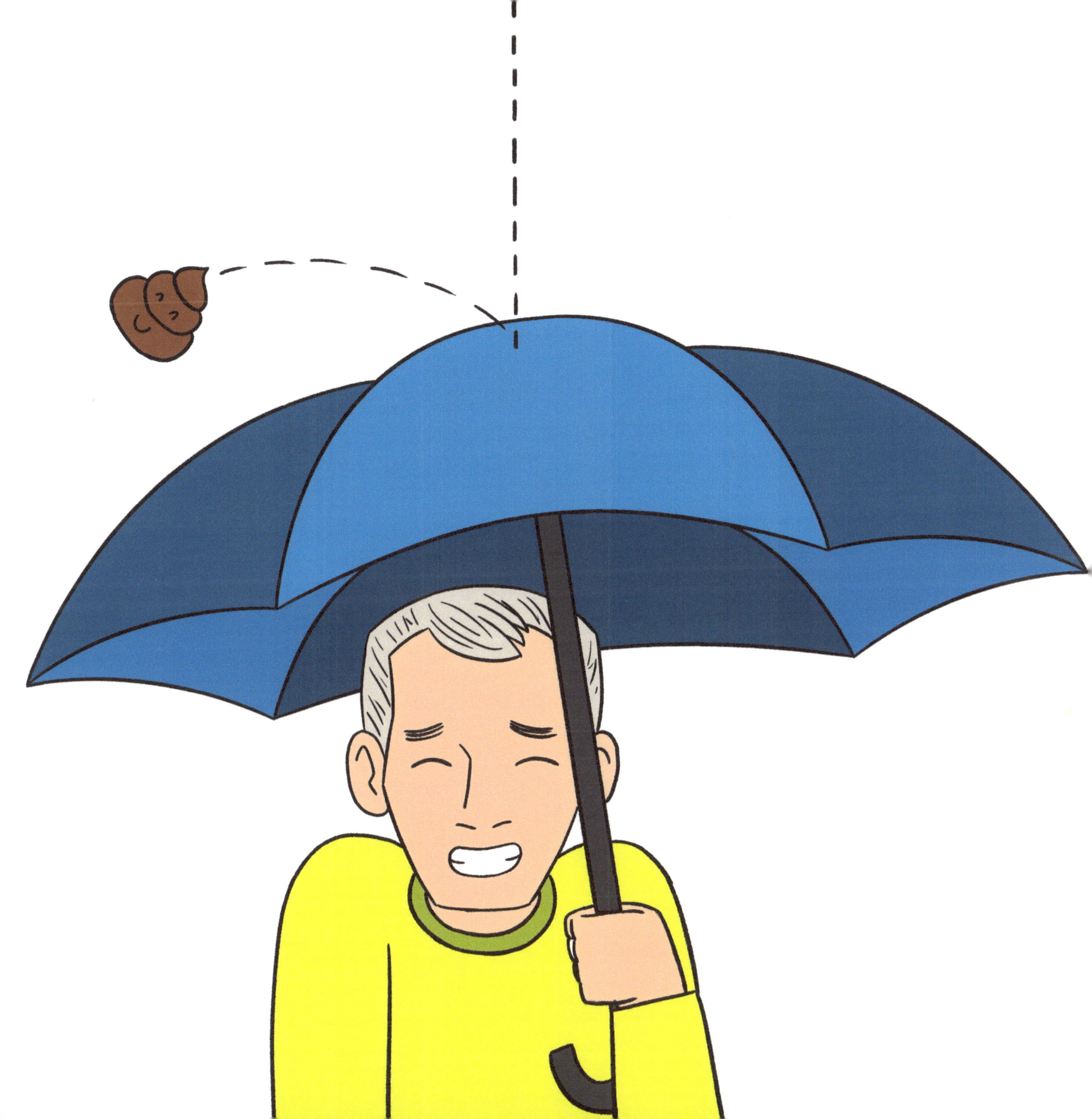

If you're 45 or older,
And scared to get this done.
Then bring along a friend,
And now it's twice as fun.

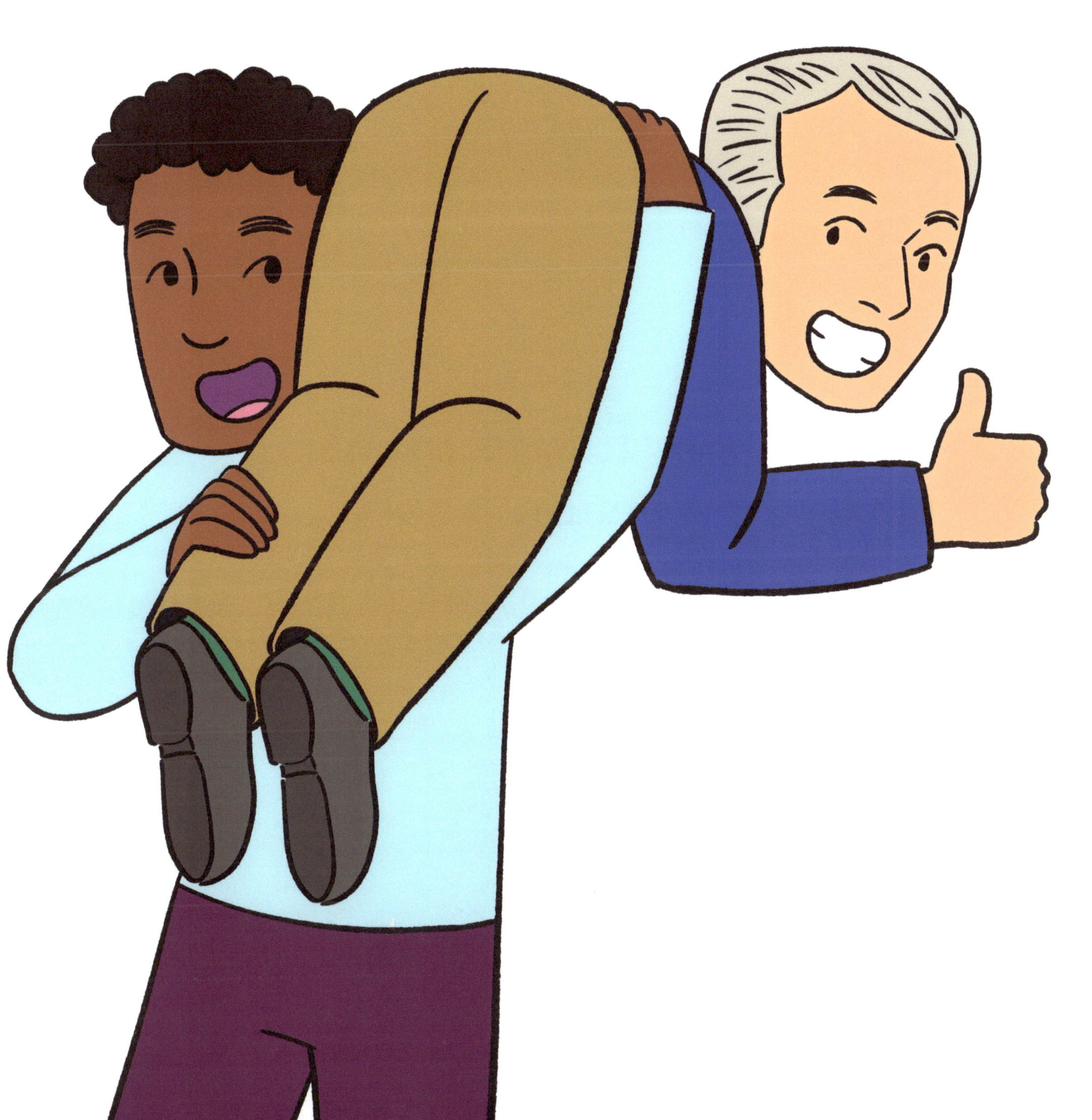

If you have future plans,
Or even a vision board.
Go call up your doctor,
And go get your butt explored.

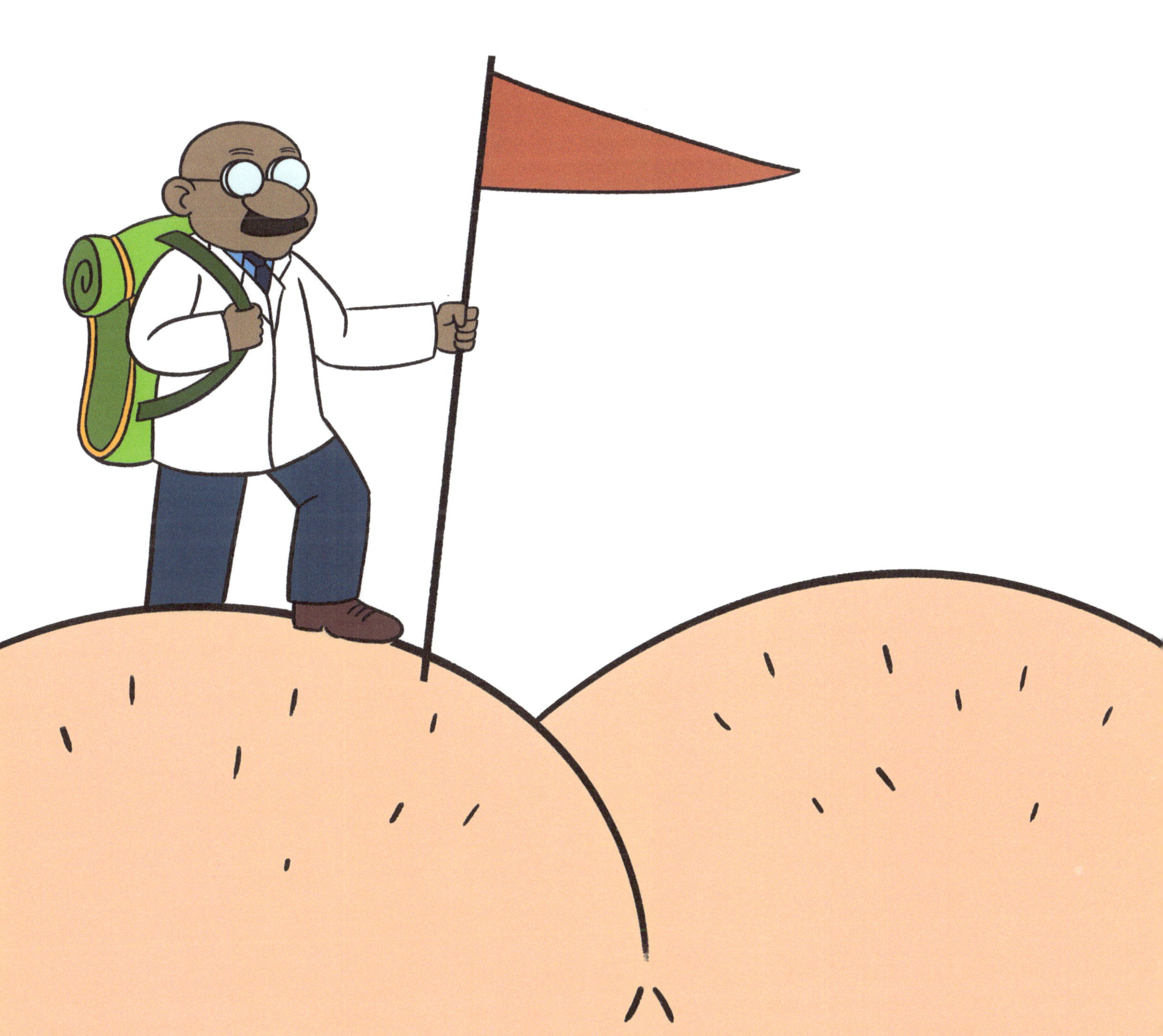

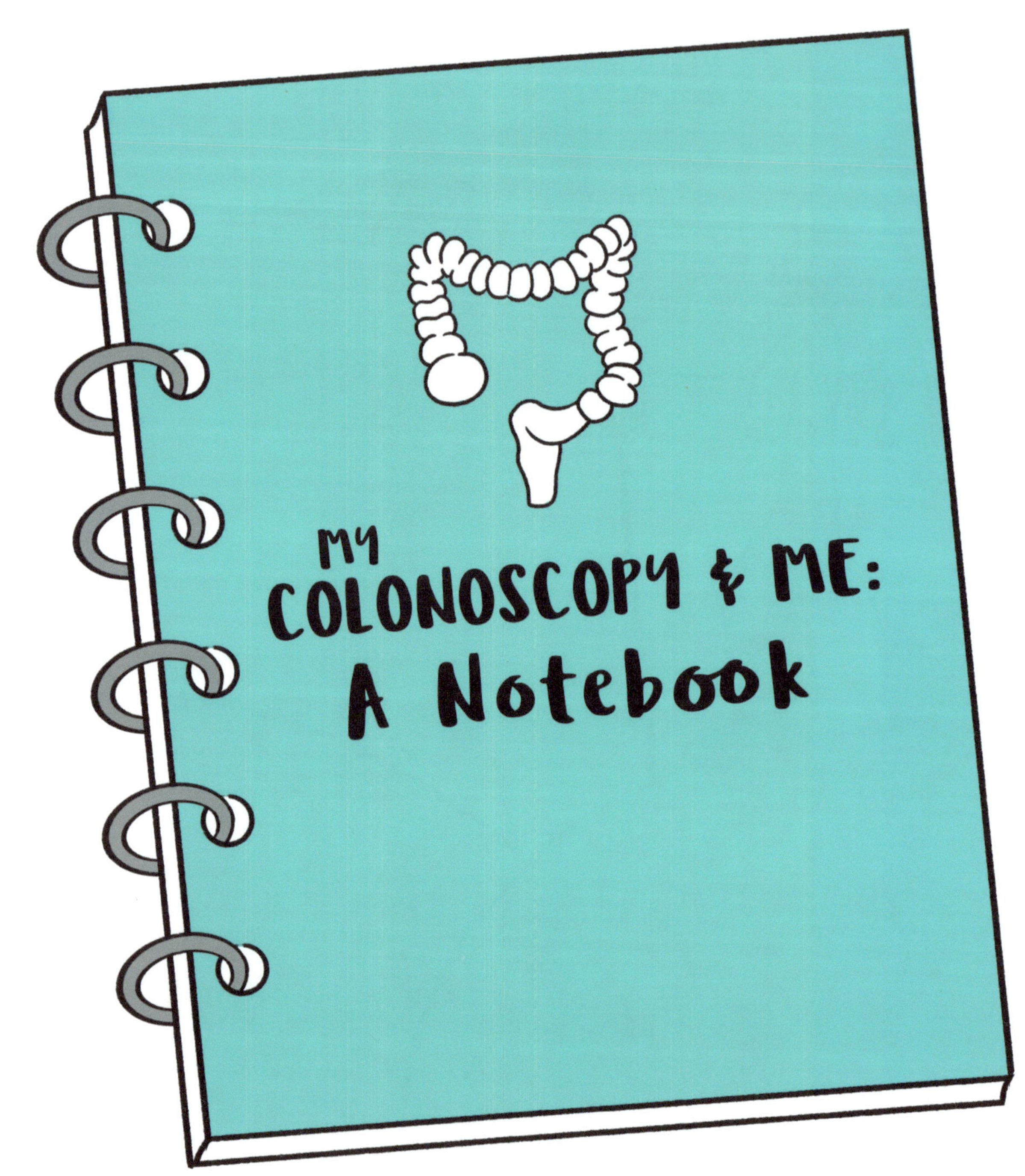

MY
COLONOSCOPY & ME:
A Notebook

UPCOMING EXAM

Date & Time: ___________________________

Doctor: ___________________________

Driver: ___________________________

Results: ___________________________

____

____

____

Notes: ___________________________

____

____

Next Exam Period: ___________________________

UPCOMING EXAM

Date & Time: _______________________________

Doctor: _______________________________

Driver: _______________________________

Results: _______________________________

____

____

____

Notes: _______________________________

____

____

Next Exam Period: _______________________________

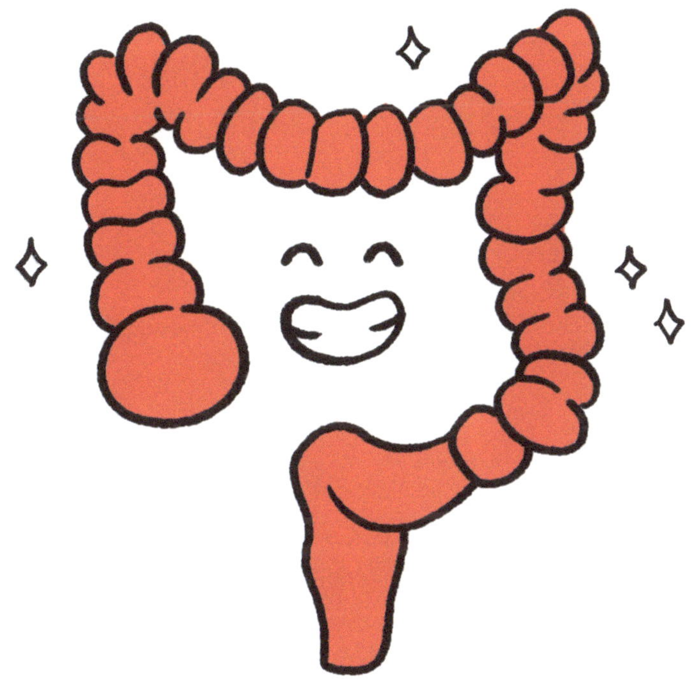